O'Brien's Radiology

for the
Ambulatory Equine Practitioner

Timothy R. O'Brien
DVM, PhD, DACVR
Professor
University of California-Davis
School of Veterinary Medicine
Department of Surgical and
Radiological Sciences
Davis, California

T0132733

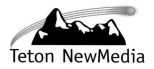

Teton NewMedia

Jackson, Wyoming
www.veterinarywire.com

Executive Editor: Carroll C. Cann
Development Editor: Susan L. Hunsberger
Design and Layout: Sue Haun 5640 Design www.fiftysixforty.com
Production Manager: Mike Albiniak 5640 Design www.fiftysixforty.com

Teton NewMedia
P.O. Box 4833
4125 South Hwy 89, Suite 1
Jackson, WY 83001

1-888-770-3165
veterinarywire.com
tetonnewmedia.com

Printed in the United States of America

ISBN# 1-59161014-1

Print Number 5 4 3 2 1

Preface

The scope of equine radiology is broad, encompassing radiography and radiographic interpretation. Although there are a number of textbooks in these areas, in my opinion these books have inadequately covered the field of diagnostic radiology in optimum breadth and depth for the equine practitioner, veterinary student, and equine resident. Consequently, this book was produced to satisfy the need, as I see it, for a definitive text in equine diagnostic radiology: one that sufficiently reflects and reinforces the instruction I currently consider appropriate for a veterinary curriculum. The information in this text is based on my lecture notes and information used for laboratory instruction. My experiences from the classroom, practice laboratories, and in clinical rotations have provided a unique understanding of the important information needed by a veterinarian to detect and understand radiographic signs necessary to establish a differential diagnosis.

There are three important factors that stimulated me to write this textbook. Two of these are the inadequacies of veterinary education and the rapid development in the last decade of imaging modalities available to the equine practitioner.

Diagnostic radiology is the backbone of imaging performed by the equine practitioner. Veterinary education in North America consists on average of between three and four hours of equine radiology lectures during the four years of the veterinary medical education. Additionally, the university diagnostic radiologist must provide a broad educational experience to students covering the areas of small animal radiology, diagnostic ultrasound, magnetic resonance imaging (MRI), computed tomography (CT), nuclear medicine, and therapeutic radiology. There are very few radiologists with a primary interest in equine diagnostic radiology.

The second important factor that stimulated me to produce this textbook has been the rapid expansion of the radiological sciences resulting in additional information available to the equine practitioner. Diagnostic radiology has provided valuable interpretative information to the equine practitioner for decades. This modality remains the primary means of imaging available to most equine practitioners. Diagnostic radiology provides information related primarily to bone and joint diseases plus limited soft tissue interpretation. Diagnostic ultrasound that is available to equine practitioners allows more extensive soft tissue evaluation particularly the detailed assessment of tendons and ligaments suspected to have sustained injury. Nuclear medical procedures (scintigraphy) have been introduced and have an advantage of permitting identification of areas of bone and joint disease before changes can be identified with diagnostic radiology. MRI and CT have been introduced permitting better and more complete lesion detection and assessment. Finally, digital imaging has recently become available to equine practitioners permitting manipulation of image quality plus electronic transfer and storage of images.

These areas of expansion of the radiological sciences are expensive and require additional training to utilize them effectively. Their introduction and use do not eliminate the need for expertise in diagnostic radiology.

These factors, plus my retirement from an active teaching role after 35 years at the University, resulted in my goal of providing a text covering radiography and basic interpretative information for the equine practitioner. This text does not include evaluation of the head, spine, thorax, abdomen, and the proximal fore and hind limbs. It is concentrated in the anatomical regions where most equine practitioners can produce diagnostic radiographs and there is a frequent clinical need for radiographic examinations; i.e., the carpus and the stifle and distally to the foot.

This text is without references. The information presented includes ideas and writings by many that have been documented or modified through my clinical experience. I apologize to my predecessors and contemporaries, both known and unknown, for this exclusion, but this text was developed as a practical teaching aid for the equine-oriented student and practitioner. It represents my belief that the information is accurate and represents the 2004 state of our knowledge base.

There will be times when a reader concludes the information I have presented is incorrect. This is certainly a possibility. I challenge that reader to document my error(s) and publish the correction. This response will result in improvement of our knowledge base . . . a benefit to all.

My special gratitude is expressed to several individuals for their contributions to this text.

To **John Neves** and **David Benzick** for their valuable technical work and insights related to equine radiography, and especially John who worked with me for 30 years as the chief equine radiographer. John helped develop several special radiographic views, and he also provided numerous editorial comments about this text.

To **Drs. Sarah Puchalski**, **Angela Hartman**, **Eric Johnson**, **Megan Richie**, and **David Detweiler**, residents who read the chapters in draft form and contributed many valuable suggestions, and especially Dr. Richie for her detailed critique throughout the production phases of this book.

To **John Doval** whose outstanding expertise and creativity transformed my rough sketches and images into highly informative illustrations and photographs. These services have significantly contributed to the value of this book.

To **Dianne Neri** who provided numerous services in the preparation of the text including typing, proofreading, and keeping the workflow organized and moving forward.

Finally, to the **past equine-oriented students and residents at the University of California and equine practitioners in general** who taught me the need to explain both what to look for and the variations that can occur in the radiographic manifestation of disease processes.

To all of you I say a sincere, "**Thank You.**"

Dedication

To my wife, Janet, for all her love and support. To my children, Shawn and Michael, my daughter-in-law, Yumi, and my grandchildren, Christina and Kelly; thank you for always being there for me.

Finally to my parents, Bill and Peg and my brother Billy Lee, for their memories and guidance.

My thanks to all of you for sharing my life.

Glossary

AEP	Ambulatory Equine Practitioner
AOE	Annual Operating Expenses
CC View	Caudocranial View
CDE Tendon	Common Digital Extensor Tendon
CR	Computed Radiography
DDF Tendon	Deep Digital Flexor Tendon
DEE	Distal Extremity Examination
DFB	Distal Flexor Border of the Navicular Bone
DHWT	Doral Hoof Wall Thickness
DI	Digital Imaging
DIJ	Distal Interphalangeal Joint
DIT Joint	Distal Intertarsal Joint
DOD	Developmental Orthopedic Disease
DPI View	Dorsoplantar View
DR	Direct or Digital Radiography
DX°Pr-PaDiO	Descriptive terminology for how a radiographic view can be produced using simple angulation. This term describes the locations of the x-ray tube (DX°Pr) and the cassette (PaDi) for producing an oblique radiograph.
DX°PrY°M(L)-PaDiL(M)O	Descriptive terminology for how both the lateral and medial oblique views can be produced using compound angulation (see Chapter 5:II-2B).
EP	Extensor Process of P3
E-STS	Extracapsular – Soft Tissue Swelling
IA	Infectious Arthritis
I-STS	Intracapsular – Soft Tissue Swelling
LDE Tendon	Lateral Digital Extensor Tendon
MO and LO	Medial and lateral oblique views. The dorsal contour silhouetted on a radiographic view that is identified, i.e., the MO highlights the dorsomedial aspect of the area.
ND	Navicular Disease
PIJ	Proximal Interphalangeal Joint
PIT Joint	Proximal Intertarsal Joint
PNBG	Periosteal New Bone Growth
SDF Tendon	Superficial Digital Flexor Tendon
SJD	Secondary Joint Disease
STS	Soft Tissue Swelling
TMT Joint	Tarsometatarsal Joint

Contents

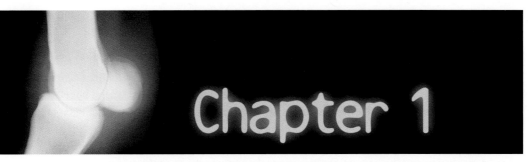

Producing High Quality Radiographs

I. Introduction

The subject dealing with the ambulatory equine practitioner (AEP) producing high quality radiographs is extensive. I have decided to present it in conjunction with the distal extremity examination (DEE) because producing high quality DEE radiographs is key for the successful equine practitioner. I conclude this based on four reasons: The DEE is one of the most important radiographic examinations the equine practitioner must perform; disorders of the foot are common causes of equine lameness encountered in clinical practice; the clinical examination of the foot is often inconclusive and the results can be relatively nonspecific; and the DEE is an extremely important part of most purchase examinations.

Performing a routine DEE is difficult work. This is because the horse is often wearing shoes at the time of the examination, the foot may be dirty, and patient cooperation can be less than satisfactory. On the positive side, most lesions occur in certain regions on a given bone resulting in a relatively easy diagnosis with high quality radiographs.

Improving the quality of your DEE will increase one's diagnostic accuracy and allow more effective treatment of a variety of disease processes affecting the equine digit. This will help make a more accurate prognosis and result in a greater degree of professional satisfaction.

However, one must have adequate equipment to produce high quality radiographs. For the AEP, this includes the X-ray machine, imaging system, and related accessory items.

1. X-Ray Unit

There are a limited number of companies producing machines for the AEP and the number of companies has decreased in the last five years. Four suppliers of units are Bowie, Medison, MinXray, and Sternes. There has been a trend to develop high frequency (HF) units because greater exposure capabilities can be achieved with units of less weight. MinXray produces three such units, i.e., the HF80+ (21 pounds), the HF8015 ultralight (14 pounds), and the HF 100/30 ultralight (27 pounds).

A. Purchasing an X-Ray Unit

It is important to emphasize certain points for veterinarians considering the purchase of an X-ray unit.
1) Purchase a new unit, not a used unit.
2) Purchase a unit that you can get serviced quickly and effectively.
3) Expect units to weigh less and be more efficient in the future.
4) Expect a 10-15% discount from the manufacturer suggested retail price (MSRP) and greater discounts may be available if multiple units are purchased.
5) Determine the service record for suppliers of units in your geographical location. Reliable service and a fast turn-around time are a necessity for the AEP. This information can often best be determined by consulting with other practitioners at local or regional meetings. These consultations may also result in the determination of others interested in purchasing a new unit leading to group purchases and greater discounts noted in 4) One can also ask dealers to provide a reference list of who has purchased a unit in your area.

Other considerations in your purchase are:
6) Does the unit have a light beam collimator and sturdy carrying case.
7) A stand is a legal requirement and varies in cost from $300 (tripod) to $2,000 (Figure 1-1).

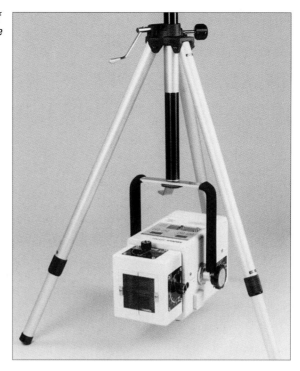

Figure 1-1. *A tripod stand best meets the needs of the AEP for holding the portable x-ray unit because it is the least expensive, light weight, and more easily stored for travel than other x-ray stands.*

The last point for consideration is which unit should be purchased. Several units can meet the needs of the AEP and the points of consideration for a purchase I have made are extremely important. However, based on experiences in our practice, the MinXray HF8015 ultralight is highly recommended for the AEP because it is very reliable, lightweight, easy to use, and we have had timely service when needed.

B. Preventing Damage to an X-Ray Unit
Damage to the X-ray unit of the AEP must be minimized because the X-ray unit is expensive representing about 40% of the fixed costs for radiography. A few tips for preventing damage to your unit include:
1) Avoid improper line voltage.
2) Secure the unit during transport.
3) Do not "over" extend the power cord.
4) Do not pound on the keypad.
5) Do not set the unit down and leave it next to a horse between exposures.

Improper line voltage can be rectified by purchasing an inexpensive line voltage measuring unit. A unit can be purchased in many electronic specialty retail stores for approximately twenty-five dollars. The tip dealing with "over" extending the power cord relates to the AEP trying to make a six-foot power cord stretch another "few" inches. This is a common problem that the AEP must avoid.

2. Imaging Systems
The advent of rare earth screens and film has been a great benefit to equine radiography. These imaging systems permit high quality radiography using the portable x-ray unit because they are much faster than the traditional calcium tungstate systems (rare earth systems have an energy conversion approximately four times calcium tungstate systems). In addition, they are less

sensitive to scatter radiation in the diagnostic range of exposure factors used by the AEP. This effect eliminates the need for a grid when doing radiograph examinations including and distal to the carpus and stifle.

A. Background Information

Rare earth intensifying screens have a MSRP of approximately $2.85/square inch independent of the speed. Screens are described as fine, medium, regular, and fast, depending on the size of the phosphor. Rather than describe the different company's products, I will provide tips and information the AEP needs to know.

1) The speed of an imaging system is given a number. This number describes the speed of the rare earth system relative to a par speed calcium tungstate system which is given a number of either 1 or 100. A "400" speed system is four times that for the par speed calcium tungstate system, and it is the recommended speed for the AEP.

2) The color of the light emitted by the screens must be the same color to which the film is sensitive, i.e., green emitting screens and green light sensitive film or blue emitting screens with blue light sensitive film.

3) If the screens emit one color and the film is sensitive to another color of light, the speed of the system will be reduced at least by a factor of two.

4) The color of light emitted by the screen can be determined by exposing the screen of an open cassette to an x-ray beam in a dark room and observing the color of light emitted.

5) Deals can be made when purchasing imaging systems.

B. Suggestions Concerning Rare Earth Imaging Systems

The subject of imaging systems is extensive. However, I have summarized some suggestions about film-screen combinations that are important for the AEP:

1) Be consistent in the film you use once your imaging system has been established and high quality radiographs are being produced, i.e, don't buy cheap film.

2) Keep your system simple by limiting the speeds and brands.

3) Take time to learn about your system by establishing variable exposures to enhance soft tissue versus bone. Many AEP are producing overexposed radiographs that do not permit soft tissue evaluation (Figure 1-2). The typical overexposure (time = x) needs a reduction in time by a factor of at least two (t = x/2) for both bone and soft tissue interpretation. The time should be reduced an additional factor of two (t = x/4) for additional soft tissue evaluation.

4) Examine and clean your screens regularly (often) with a good commercial screen cleaner.

5) A 400-speed imaging system is recommended for the AEP. Major producers of 400-speed systems are AGFA, Kodak, MCI OPTONIX, and 3M.

3. Cassettes

Intensifying screens are expensive and must be protected against damage by being placed within cassettes. Hard cassettes provide the AEP this protection. The MSRP for rigid cassettes are approximately $80 for an 8"x10", $100 for a 10"x12", and $180 for a 14"x17" cassette, but the prices are variable. An advantage to the hard cassette is they last for a long time if properly cared for and especially if damage is avoided. **The horse should not stand directly on the cassette.** Many hard cassettes can be re-screened giving the undamaged cassette a longer life. The disadvantage to the hard cassette for the AEP is increased weight and size (Figure 1-3). As a result, vinyl cassettes are frequently used by the AEP. Vinyl cassettes are not new. They were used decades ago. However, their use with rare earth screens has more recently been developed by 3M. In summary, the vinyl cassette is much lighter and less expensive, but they are less durable and are available only in the 8" x 10" size.

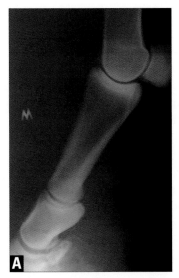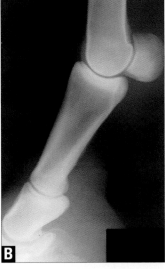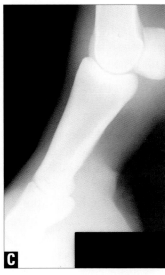

Figure 1-2. The AEP should be able to adjust exposure time for an exposure, that permits a more accurate evaluation. Over-exposure (time [t] = x) is a common problem of the AEP **(A)** that can be corrected by reducing the exposure time **(B)** by a factor of two (t=x/2). Further time reduction by a factor of two (t=x/4) permits soft tissue and periosteal interpretation to be maximized **(C)**.

An often-asked question deals with used cassettes. If one is considering used cassettes, be sure they are light-proof and not damaged. The cost to recondition a cassette must be determined and integrated into the decision to utilize used cassettes. In addition, it is highly likely the used cassettes will need re-screening.

If in doubt about purchasing used hard cassettes, it is recommended to get new cassettes. If cost prevents the purchase of new cassettes, then investigate the program 3M has for vinyl cassettes.

Finally, there is the question of how many cassettes are recommended for the AEP. This question is difficult to answer because it varies with the practice demands, working environment, and finances. The same is true for the size(s) of the cassettes. However, I recommend at least ten 8"x10" cassettes with rare earth screens for the AEP who does a significant amount of lameness work in the field.

Figure 1-3. A comparison of nine hard and vinyl cassettes show the difference in size and space required for these types of cassettes. The vinyl cassette holder can be seen under the stack of vinyl cassettes. The vinyl cassettes are available only in the 8"x10" size.

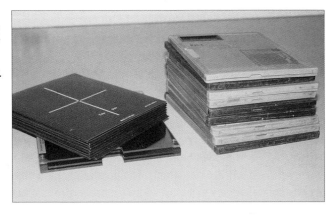

4. Digital Imaging (DI)

Radiography has made the leap from analog (film-screen) to digital systems resulting in benefits for image quality manipulation, storage, and sending images electronically. Digital radiography (DR) systems are on the market providing larger image receptors, higher resolution, and increased functionality. Lower prices are expected for these systems as competition and innovation develop. The DI modes are referred to as DR (direct radiography) and CR (computed radiography). The two are distinguished by DR being cassetteless and CR being cassette-based. DR is faster for producing readable images because CR requires each cassette to be placed in a cassette reader before the image is sent to the computer to produce an image. Digital imaging has the primary advantages to the AEP in an ability to manipulate and enhance image quality and to send digital images via the internet. The major disadvantage is digital imaging requires a substantial investment (currently in the six figures) to purchase a system. Most AEP will not be able to afford these systems because the radiography volume does not make them cost effective. Most digital imaging systems currently being purchased for equine radiology are being placed in academic institutions and large group practices. However, this technology is expected to become widely used as the cost becomes more affordable for small groups of AEPs.

5. Related Items Needed to Produce High Quality Radiographs

As indicated at the beginning, the distal extremity examination will be incorporated into this presentation. Needed for the distal extremity and other examinations are foot preparation items, identification techniques, positioning aides, safety equipment, and a means to process exposed film. Most of the expenses associated with these items are provided in Economic Issues of Radiology for the AEP, Chapter 2.

A. Foot Preparation

The shoe should be removed and the foot cleaned and packed before radiographs of the DEE are taken. Failure to do so is probably the most common cause of a non-diagnostic DEE (cannot be accurately interpreted). To properly prepare the equine foot for radiographic examination, the following items are required:

1) Shoe removal equipment.
2) Hoof pick, knife, and rasp.
3) Heavy scrub brush, soap, and plastic bucket.
4) A soft tissue equivalent density material for packing the sulci. A modeling compound works well for this, e.g., Play-Doh (Tonka Corp, Pawtucket, RI).
5) A two- to three-foot square of heavy canvas. The canvas is necessary for the horse to stand upon after the foot has been packed, and it is also used to wrap the other items for the foot examination during storage.

B. Radiographic Identification

Imprinting tape or a light flasher system. This is needed to permanently identify the radiographs. The information required is the owner's name, horse's name or number, date of the radiographic examination, the name of veterinarian or hospital, and location (Figure 1-4).

Radio-opaque marking tape is commonly used by AEP for identification. Information concerning the owner, horse, and date can be simply written with a ballpoint pen and placed within your personalized holder blocker and attached to the cassette prior to exposure. The holder blocker permits the name of the veterinarian/clinic and location to be included on the radiograph and can include a LF-RF-LH-RH indicator*. The holder blockers are available in four opacity levels to accommodate various exposure settings, but it is recommended the AEP get the III (yellow)

* X-Rite, Grandville, MI (Style 178A) or MED I.D., Grand Rapids, MI (Style 204D)

O'Brien's Equine Service
(530) 123-4567, Box 123, Davis, CA 95616

Case # ______________________ Date __________

Owner ________________________________

Horse ______________________ Sex __________

Breed ______________________ Age __________

Figure 1-4. *The identification information permanently recorded on a radiograph should include the names of the owner and horse, date of the radiographic examination, and the name and location of the veterinarian. Other beneficial information includes details on the patient and the veterinarian's telephone number.*

density levels. Marking tape can be purchased in rolls or pre-cut 3" strips. It is recommended that the AEP purchase 3/4" wide tape in the Mini-Pak (100 strips).

Positioning identification. Radiodense markers are for location identification and include:

a. Right and left
b. Front and hind
c. Medial and lateral
d. Non-weight bearing and partial weight bearing

Other identification materials:

a. For the outer surface of the dorsal hoof wall, e.g., wire, solder, or barium paste.
b. For a draining skin wound, bump or lump, BB's are taped to the area for this identification function prior to the radiographic examination.

C. Positioning Aides

1) Cassette Tunnel: The horse should **never** have its foot on a cassette when weight bearing. Tunnels are available to accommodate the 8"x10" hard cassette (Figure 1-5). The vinyl cassette tunnel is seen in Figure 1-3 under the vinyl cassettes. The top should be clear for visualization of the cassette and the top is made out of special polycarbonate material (not plexiglass).
2) Slotted Positioning Block: The block is made from hard wood with a 7/8-inch wide slot cut at a 65° angle from horizontal (Figure 1-6). This slot is wide enough to hold a 9/16-inch hard cassette. This permits repeatable 45° DP (Dorso45° proximal-palmarodistal oblique)

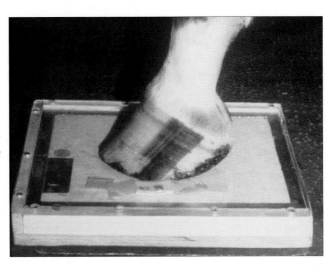

Figure 1-5. *A cassette tunnel for the hard cassette provides protection against cassette damage for three views taken as part of the routine DEE. Note the cassette blocker can be seen through the clear polycarbonate top, identification markers are included, and a thin sheet of lead has been positioned under the tunnel to minimize backscatter from the concrete floor.*

projections to be made, and the block is used for the LM projection. The cassette tunnel is used for the other three projections of the DEE.

3) Cassette Holder: An aluminum 8"x10" cassette holder with interchangeable handles is needed for positioning and radiation safety. The short handle (12 inches) seems more convenient for the AEP than the long handle (30 inches).

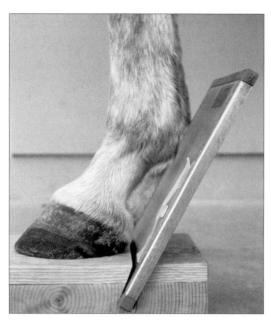

Figure 1-6. *The slotted wooden block is a positioning aide for producing the 45°DP and lateromedial projections.*

4) Laser Pointer: A small laser pointer can be purchased and attached to the X-ray tube head of most units (not the MinXray HF8015 ultralight) for localization of the central beam while positioning. This is beneficial but the cost is approximately $650.

5) Reddin Positioning Device: This item is designed to control the distance between the tube head and cassette. It replaces a measuring device but costs approximately $250. It has been described by some AEP as being cumbersome to work with and store for travel in the vehicle.

D. Radiation Safety

This is an extremely important topic for the AEP, but it is extensive and often the AEP has limited interest in this topic. Therefore, I will summarize some very important points about radiation safety.

1) The veterinarian producing the radiographic examination is responsible for all radiation safety issues during the procedure.

2) Radiation exposures to yourself and staff must be monitored. Film badges are recommended for monitoring rather than pencil dosimeters, because the readings on the film badge are a source for a permanent record.

3) Safety equipment must be provided including:
   a. Lead gloves with fingers (2 pairs)
   b. Lead aprons (2)
   c. Aluminum cassette holder

Safety equipment is designed to protect personnel from scatter radiation, not the primary beam. In addition, the best protection from radiation exposure is distance. The gloves and aprons have 0.5 mm lead equivalent and are actually rubberized tin. It is important to emphasize that body parts of the veterinarian, staff, or clients **must not be within the primary beam**. This especially includes unprotected fingers used to hold the cassette.

4) Optional safety equipment for those closest to the exposure field:
   a. Leaded safety glasses (2 pairs)
   b. Leaded neck collar for thyroid protection (1)

E. Film Processing

The AEP has three general options for processing exposed film including purchasing a tabletop unit, a rebuilt large unit, or establishing creative techniques.

1) Tabletop Processor - There are several brands of these units and the cost will be related to the brand. These units generally will have a cost range of $4,200 – 6,500.

2) Rebuilt Large Processor – This is a good way to solve your processing needs if your volume is great enough. Kodak units seem to be the best for cost and function. A 90-second rebuilt Kodak processor should cost $6,000 – 8,000 with the capability of producing 500 8"x10" radiographs per hour. (Note: A new processor could be considered as a fourth option but the cost at approximately $29,000 makes it a less likely option for the AEP.)

3) Creative Solutions to Processing – The AEP commonly uses other facilities including human and veterinary hospitals. This option works best when the volume of processing is not great. Human hospitals seem to be an excellent source for processing and the cost is variable. Many AEPs have reported this service is free because they provide incentives (donuts, etc) to the technical staff, and the physician radiologists enjoy looking at the radiographs of horses because they are so different. Other human and veterinary facilities use a charge/radiograph fee.

II. Radiographic Quality

A goal of this chapter is to provide a broad background so you will be able to improve the radiographic quality in your practice resulting in a more accurate radiographic diagnosis. Errors in interpretation often occur due to correctable technical problems. Radiographic quality errors are diverse, but I have capsulated, according to their point of origin, those of the equine practitioners as preparation, production, and processing, or the three "P's." The most common quality errors and their causes are:

1. Lack of Proper Foot Preparation
   A. Not removing the shoe
   B. Inadequate cleaning of the foot
   C. Improper packing of the sulci

2. Production Errors
   A. Improper exposure factors
   B. Poor radiographic positioning
   C. Inadequate number of views
   D. Motion artifacts: Sedation is commonly used so a quality radiographic examination can be performed. The following intravenous medications are used in my practice for shorter and longer periods of sedation for the average-sized adult horse. For shorter term sedation, xylazine[1] is administered at a dosage of 150-200 mg (0.2-0.3 mg/kg). For longer term sedation, detomidine[2] is used at 3-5 mg (6-10 µg/kg). In those horses that are apprehensive following either xylazine or detomidine, butorphanol[3] is given at a dose of 3-5 mg (6-10 µg/kg).

[1] Vedco, St. Joseph, MO [2] Pfizer Animal Health, Exton, PA [3] Fort Dodge, IA

3. Processing or Darkroom Problems

    A. Inadequate temperature control of chemical solutions
    B. Poor darkroom chemistry
    C. Darkroom exposure problems
    D. Dirty or wet hands and rough handling of film
    E. Not using a safelight with proper filtration

Excellent radiographic quality is the goal each equine practitioner must be interested in attaining. Assume your radiographs are classified as either "poor quality" or "needs improvement." How can one improve the quality of radiographs?

4. Sources Responsible for Poor Quality

Quality error(s) may result from problems in preparation, production, and processing. The most difficult problem for the AEP to determine is whether a production or processing problem is occurring.

    A. Production errors are attributed to the X-ray machine, imaging system, and examination techniques. X-ray machine-related problems result from exposure factors (mAs and kVp) and focal-film distance (FFD) variation. Common imaging system problems are improper screen-film matching or worn-out (or damaged) screens. Examination technique problems result from improper foot preparation, poor positioning, inadequate radiographic identification, or insufficient number of projections. My experiences indicate the more common problems are variation in FFD (Figure 1-7), worn-out screens, improper foot preparation, or inadequate number of projections.

    B. Processing errors depend on whether manual or automatic processing is utilized. Manual processing tends to lead to more quality problems than occurs with a regularly serviced automatic processor. Chemical problems are often attributed to the use of outdated or improperly diluted developer or fixer. Temperature control and timing problems during processing often occur, but film fog due to improper darkroom lighting is also common. This includes safe lights and exterior lighting. The solution to most of these processing errors is proper darkroom maintenance and/or an automatic processor. Automatic processor requires the careful monitoring of the chemical levels (especially the fixer) when not used on a daily basis. Evaporation of the fixer occurs more rapidly than the developer.

5. Improving Your Radiographic Quality!

A practical solution to determine whether poor quality is due to darkroom or production problems can be the utilization of a clinical or hospital facility (veterinary or human) that does a large volume of high quality radiography. Load a cassette and immediately produce an exposure of any anatomical area using your technique for the selected projection. Empty the cassette and reload it with identical film. Make a second exposure of the same anatomical area with identical exposure factors, including distance. Process one exposed film in your facility and the other in the clinic or hospital (human or veterinary) that produces high quality radiographs.

    A. If the radiograph processed at the other hospital is of high quality compared with the one processed at your facility, then it is a processing problem rather than a production problem.

    B. A poor quality radiograph from both facilities indicates a production problem.

Another available remedy for poor radiographic quality is to hire an x-ray technologist to solve your problems. These individuals may be found at human hospitals, veterinary hospitals, or university teaching hospitals. If you need help purchasing equipment or with radiography problems and prefer to deal with someone familiar with AEP radiography, you can contact Mr. John Neves at 424 Grande Avenue, Davis, CA, 95616 (530/756-8816).

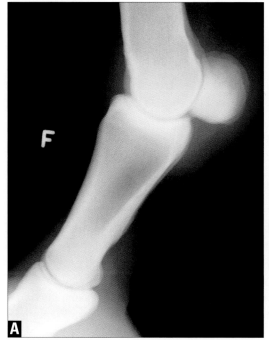

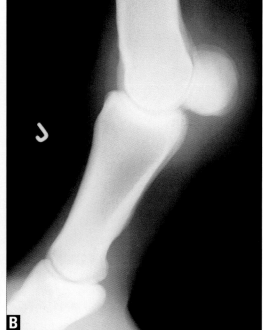

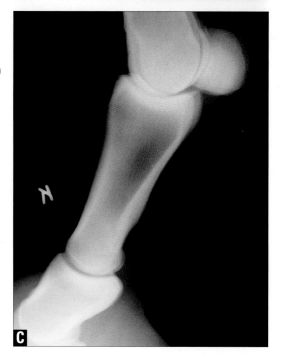

Figure 1-7. *A common source of variation in radiographic quality is produced by inconsistent focal-film distance (FFD). An exposure made at the FFD used for a routine examination (**A**) can be compared when the FFD was increased 10 percent (**B**) and decreased 10 percent (**C**). The slight minification of C is a photographic artifact.*

6. Critique for Radiographic Quality

The previous sections describe the factors contributing to a diagnostic quality radiographic examination. The application of this information will re-enforce it. A referral radiographic examination of the distal extremity was recently sent to me for interpretation. This examination provides a good opportunity to apply the information I have presented. Examine the radiographs and determine the quality of the examination before interpreting the radiographs and establishing your

Conclusions and Impressions (Figure 1-8A, B). Your critique for diagnostic quality should evaluate:
  A. Proper Foot Preparation
  B. Production Factors
     1) Exposure
     2) Positioning
     3) Number of views
  C. Processing
  D. Other Factors

III. Conclusion

The quality of medicine practiced by an AEP is directly related to the ability to produce high quality radiographic examinations! This conclusion is based on the premise that more successful treatment results from an accurate diagnosis, and high quality radiographs permit the AEP to establish a more accurate diagnosis. The second conclusion based on years of experience is that the AEP can produce high quality radiographs using a portable X-ray unit, a rare earth imaging system, and a good darkroom facility. Accessory items are important in making the radiographs diagnostic especially for the DEE. The AEP must then use proper exposure factors, take a sufficient number of projections for routine examinations, and remember to take special radiographic views to more completely evaluate an anatomical location for structural changes compatible with the differential diagnosis. Chapter 4 will provide the AEP with greater background on how to perform a routine DEE and the special views that compliment the routine radiographic examination.

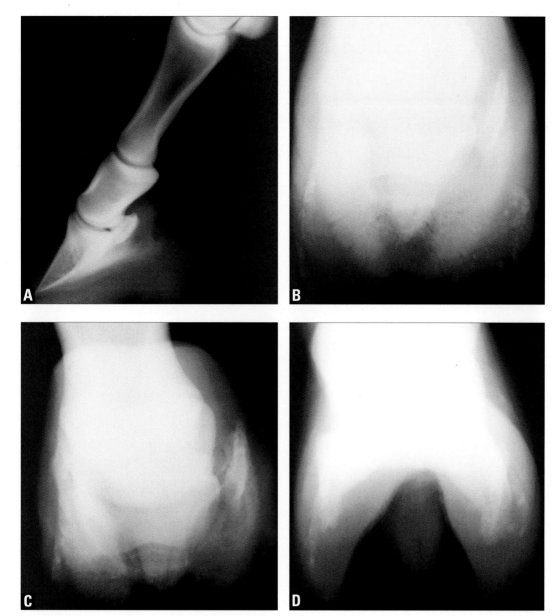

Figure 1-8A. Critique the radiographic quality of this DEE.
Figure 1-8B. The critique revealed the following:
1. Foot preparation: The shoe was removed but there was inadequate cleaning and there was an absence of packing of the sulci of the frog *(A-D)* resulting in artifacts.
2. Production factors:
Exposure: The 65°DP (C) was underexposed and wasn't coned-down so the navicular bone cannot be evaluated.
Positioning: The navicular bone cannot be seen on the flexor skyline view (D). The exposure was made with too steep a proximal angulation and there was inadequate palmar extension of the distal extremity.
Number of views: There are inadequate views for a distal extremity examination (DEE). A 45°DP projection was not included[4].
3. Processing: Processing did not contribute to a reduction in diagnostic quality.
4. Other factors: There is an absence of markers for identification. One cannot determine if this examination is of the right or left front or hind foot. In addition, medial cannot be differentiated from the lateral on the dorsopalmar (front) or dorsoplantar (hind) *(B and C)* and flexor skyline *(D)* views.
Conclusion: This referral DEE is of insufficient quality to be diagnostic, so an accurate interpretation and appropriate Conclusions and Impressions cannot be established.

[4] Chapter 4 will explain production of the DEE.

NOTES

NOTES

NOTES

Chapter 2

Economic Issues of Radiology for the Ambulatory Equine Practitioner

I. Introduction

The expenses and income associated with doing radiology as an ambulatory equine practitioner (AEP) are subjects that have received little attention in veterinary literature or in the educations of students while receiving their veterinary medical training. Consequently, few AEPs can provide an answer to the following three questions:
  1. How much does it cost you to produce an 8" x 10" radiograph?
  2. How much profit do you make for each 8" x 10" radiograph produced?
  3. What effect does the quantity of radiographs produced have on the net income you generate?

I am going to provide the methodology needed to answer these questions in a generic manner. The details I am going to present are not absolute. So, please do not try to find "errors" in this data. Rather, try to understand the methodology. **Then, apply this methodology to your practice circumstances and determine how much it costs to produce an 8" x 10" radiograph, your income, and how a greater number of radiographic examinations produced influences your net annual income**[1]. This information will be extremely valuable. In fact, when presenting this subject to AEPs, I tell them this new knowledge will allow them to reach the goal of my presentation, i.e., provide information and insights that will at least allow you to pay your expenses to attend that conference… and one more meeting each year for the foreseeable future.

To accomplish that goal, some assumptions must be made. The primary assumption is either your radiographic quality needs a lot of improvement or you are a recent graduate who does not have the equipment necessary to provide diagnostic quality radiographs. Therefore, equipment and supplies will need to be purchased. **Practitioners may have some equipment so that variables must be taken into account as one applies this methodology to one's practice circumstances.**

II. Basic Radiography Information

1. Equipment
The major equipment needed is a radiographic unit. The number of brands of portable units available to the AEP has been reduced in the last five years and now there are only four or five brands that meet the needs for most AEP. The unit one purchases should be powerful, lightweight, and reliable. Service availability is a major factor and must be weighed against variations in purchase price. High frequency units tend to be more powerful and represent the trend for the AEP. One should expect a 10-15% discount from the manufacturers suggested list price. The unit I will use for this example costs $7,500. All units come with a padded aluminum carrying case, and most have a light beam collimator.

2. Accessories
Units do not come with an X-ray stand, but a stand is required by law in the State of California. This law states that the unit housing cannot be handled at the time of exposure. The AEP should know that the MinXray units (HF80+, HF8015 ultralight, and HF100/30 ultralight) were tested at the VMTH-UCD and a measurable level of radiation was not detectable at the surface of the unit housing. Furthermore, the kVp, ma, and time setting produced accurate outputs for each setting. The cost of a stand varies from $300 - $2,000. A tripod costs $300, and is recommended because it is the least expensive and functionally it is the best for the AEP. A light beam collimator is important for producing high quality radiographs and is a standard component of most new units.

[1] The cost data used in this chapter represents costs effective 2004.

One should know that a light beam collimator can be added to a unit. The cost is approximately $900, and it will add four pounds to the overall weight of the unit. Other necessary accessory equipment includes a cassette holder ($115), tunnel ($65), and a foot positioning block ($45).

3. Imaging Systems

Rare earth screen-film combinations are the imaging systems of choice for the AEP for two major reasons. Rare earth imaging systems are more sensitive than calcium tungstate systems, allowing reduced exposure time. They are also less sensitive to scatter radiation at the exposure levels the AEP commonly utilizes for extremity radiographs so a grid is not needed. It is extremely important that the AEP understand that the film purchased must be sensitive to the color of light the screens emit or the images produced will be of poorer quality.

There are several manufacturers of screens but the three most commonly used are Kodak, AGFA, and 3M. The screens are classified as fine, medium, regular, and fast which relates to the crystal size of the light emitting phosphor. The above-classified screens have speeds from 100 to 1200. The cost for a screen is independent of speed and is priced at approximately $2.85 per square inch. Kiran and MCI Optonix screens are also available through many dealers at a lower cost.

4. Cassettes

The current extreme for cassettes are aluminum or plastic (hard) to vinyl (soft). The major differences are durability, weight, and cost. The suggested list prices for Kodak's aluminum and plastic cassettes are approximately $80 (8" x 10"), $100 (10" x 12"), and $180 (14" x 17"). Ten 8" x 10" rare earth screened cassettes are recommended for the AEP who does lameness evaluations as a significant part of their practice.

III. Cost of Producing Radiographs

There are fixed costs and annual operating expenses (AOE) for radiography. These are summarized below:

A. Fixed Costs: Equipment, etc. (Cost Range in Dollars)
   1. Portable X-ray unit ($7,500 – $10,500). $7,500
   2. Rare Earth Cassettes: Ten 8" x 10" ($200-$358) 2,900
   3. Lead gloves and aprons – 2 sets 500
   4. X-ray processor ($4,000 – $29,000): Rebuilt Kodak unit 8,000
   5. Cassette Holder: 8" x 10" 115
   6. Stand (tripod). 300
   7. Tunnel Cassette Holder ($65) and Slotted Positioning
      Block ($45) 110
   8. Identification Markers 35
   9. Two Bank View Box 350
   10. Bright Light 90
   11. Darkroom: Safelight ($80-$150);
      Imprinter ($125-$350); and
      Film Bin ($300) 600
   TOTAL $20,500

B. Annual Operating Expenses
   1. Processor chemicals – based on
      500 radiographs and changed
      6 times/per year $440
   2. Processor Maintenance Service ($60 – $80/month) 720
   3. 8" x 10" film: 500 sheets of Kodak or
      AGFA Quality ($136/box for single emulsion) 680
   4. Dosimetry: 2 Film Badges and Start-up Fee 158
   5. Identification of Radiographs: Imprinting Tape 30
   TOTAL $2,028

Therefore, the cost for producing 500 radiographs (100 examinations, consisting of five radiographs each) for the first year is $22,528 or the cost per radiograph is $45.06 ($22,528/500). However, the cost per radiograph over a five-year period is $12.26.

$$\left[\frac{20,500 + 5(2,028)}{5(500)} \right]$$

IV. Income from Producing Radiographs

The answer to the first of my earlier three questions is $12.26 for the conditions defined in this example. So, how much income did you receive from these 100 radiographic examinations consisting of 500 radiographs?

The charge for a radiograph will vary significantly in different geographical areas. A survey of AEPs in our geographic area revealed the client was charged an average of $20/radiograph. Therefore, the income calculations are:

Gross Income: 500 radiographs x $20 per radiograph	$10,000
Expenses: 500 radiographs x $12.26/radiograph	6,130
"Semi" net annual income	3,870
	(or $7.74/radiograph)

Flaw Alert

There are some major flaws in this income determination for the AEP, but they will vary with the practice and even the practitioner. This is why I indicated at the beginning of this chapter that the information was not absolute and asked you apply the methodology to your practice circumstances. Some flaws I want to point out are:

1. Retakes were not included. A five-view examination assumes the radiographic quality of each view was diagnostic.
2. Payment was received for every exposure you made.
3. Insurance on your equipment was not purchased.
4. You were not paid for your professional expertise and time.

Insurance for an X-ray unit against damage will cost a minimum of $500 annually.
Too few veterinarians receive remuneration for their time and expertise related to radiology. For

this example, I am going to assume you are a recent graduate and your time is worth $60 per hour. The value of your time is an important factor for you to consider as you do these calculations for yourself at a later time using this methodology. There are three parts to considering the time it costs you for radiology.

1. Production time.
2. Interpretation time.
3. Travel time.

I will assume it takes an average of 30 minutes to produce a five-view examination which includes setting up equipment, patient preparation, making the exposures, and storing the equipment. The radiographs must be interpreted which takes your time. This includes studying each radiograph and writing a report. One may need to review anatomy and other books so I recommend this be done in one's office, and on average 30 minutes will be required. Finally, a charge for travel time to produce the radiographic examination must be included. This travel time is highly variable related to geographical location, traffic patterns, etc, but 45 minutes was utilized as the average travel time for this example.

Therefore, the values for time to do the 100 examinations:

1. Production: 100 examinations at 0.5 hr x $60/hr	$3,000
2. Interpretation: 100 examinations at 0.5 hr x $60/hr	$3,000
3. Travel: 100 examinations at 0.75 hour x $60/hr	$4,500
TOTAL	$10,500

The cost of your time and a basic level of insurance are additional expenses that should be considered in determining "real" net income rather than the "semi" net income previously established.

"Semi" net annual income	$3,870
Costs for time and a minimum level of insurance	<$11,000>
"Real" net annual income from radiology	<$7,130>

You actually lost $14.26 on each radiograph you produced for the year! If the value of your time is greater than $60 per hour and you did not charge for your time, the loss is much greater.

V. The Effect of Volume on Radiology Income

The number of radiographic examinations an AEP produces can have a dramatic impact on the financial picture of one's practice. To demonstrate this effect, a comparison will be done considering an annual volume of 160 examinations (800 radiographs) and 60 examinations (300 radiographs) to the 100 examinations (500 radiographs) previously done. The fixed costs will remain essentially the same and the AOE will vary related primarily to the quantity of film used (assume a box [100 sheets] of 8" x 10" single emulsion film costs $136).

The Impact of the Number of Examinations
Performed (Radiographs) on Income

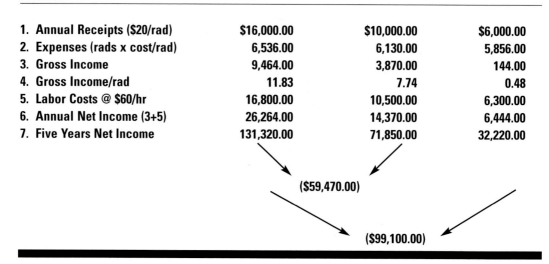

Costs	160(800)	100(500)	60(300)
1. Expenses (fixed + AOE)	$22,936.00	$22,528.00	$22,256.00
2. Cost/Radiograph for 1 year	28.67	45.06	74.19
3. Cost/Radiograph over 5 years	8.17	12.26	19.52
Differences	($4.09)	($7.26)	
	($11.35)		

Income			
1. Annual Receipts ($20/rad)	$16,000.00	$10,000.00	$6,000.00
2. Expenses (rads x cost/rad)	6,536.00	6,130.00	5,856.00
3. Gross Income	9,464.00	3,870.00	144.00
4. Gross Income/rad	11.83	7.74	0.48
5. Labor Costs @ $60/hr	16,800.00	10,500.00	6,300.00
6. Annual Net Income (3+5)	26,264.00	14,370.00	6,444.00
7. Five Years Net Income	131,320.00	71,850.00	32,220.00
	($59,470.00)		
	($99,100.00)		

Technique Criticisms

Some AEPs have critiqued these calculations and indicated some errors were made with the time calculations. These criticisms included the value of the AEP's time is too low at $60/hour, travel time should not be a part of the radiology income calculations because it is charged as part of a general ranch visit, and the time cost for production should be eliminated because it is included in the "gross income/radiograph." These are valid considerations that must be considered by the AEP as this information is applied in ones practice. The time value charge for interpretation is uncommonly made in veterinary medicine. This is true even though clients have personal exposure to an interpretation charge in human radiology. I strongly urge the submission of an interpretation charge at the least because the time of the AEP has value and shouldn't be given away. This action is justified because it will stimulate greater interest in careful interpretation, which will result in an improved evaluation of the radiographs leading to a more accurate diagnosis. The net effects will result in an increased quality of medicine practiced and it will be financially rewarding.

VI. Conclusions

Radiology can allow one to reach the goal of this presentation, i.e., ... pay for this conference (book) and one meeting each year for the foreseeable future. However, one must know:

1. Production costs for their radiographs.
2. How to produce high quality radiographs efficiently.
3. The financial impact of volume of radiographs produced.
4. To charge for one's professional expertise and time.
5. Apply the methodology used in this chapter to your practice.

It must be emphasized that the value of this information requires its application to your practice

NOTES

NOTES

NOTES

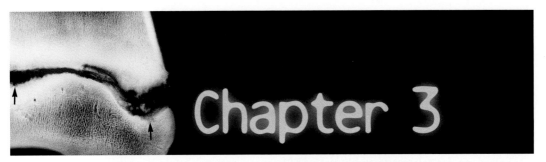

Chapter 3

Radiographic Interpretation of Horses with Clinical Signs of Infection or Joint Disease

I. Radiographic Interpretation of Soft Tissue Infection

1. Cellulitis

Radiographic evaluation of a horse with clinical signs of cellulitis is done primarily to determine the presence of a radiodense foreign body and signs of osteomyelitis. **The radiographic findings to be evaluated with cellulitis are the presence of the following:**

- **Extracapsular soft tissue swelling (E-STS)**
- **Radiodense foreign body**
- **Gas in the soft tissues (Figure 3-1)**
- **Periosteal reaction or cortical destructive change in the area of the STS**

E-STS is identified by increased density and a loss of normal soft tissue planes. Horses with chronic cellulitis often have a draining tract (Figure 3-2). These patients should have a special radiographic examination with a positive contrast agent injected into the tract. This special procedure is called "fistulography."

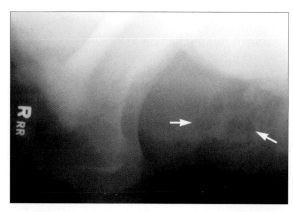

Figure 3-1. Gas within the soft tissues is one of four radiographic signs associated with a diagnosis of cellulitis. The gas seen in the tissues caudal to the stifle was produced by a gas-forming bacterial infection. Penetrating wounds, fistulous tracts, compound fractures, and iatrogenic lesions are the other causes for gas accumulations in the soft tissues.

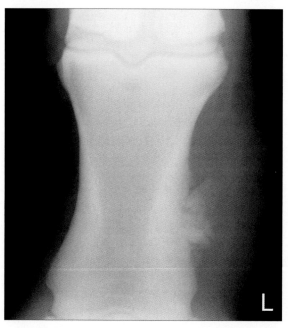

Figure 3-2. Extracapsular soft tissue swelling and a chronic periosteal reaction at the lateral aspect of distal P1 without gas in the soft tissues were identified radiographically in a horse with a chronic draining tract. The radiographic quality was enhanced by reducing the exposure time by a factor of two permitting better visualization of the soft tissues and periosteal reaction. Fistulography was indicated to evaluate for the presence of a radiolucent foreign body and to determine if the fistulous tract communicates with the chronic periosteal reaction.

2. Fistulography

Fistulography is extremely valuable in determining the cause, direction, and extent of the soft tissue tract(s) as well as identifying a lucent foreign body. Common causes of the chronic cellulitis with a draining tract are a foreign body, osteomyelitis with or without sequestration, or chronic infection.

A positive contrast agent and sterile delivery agents are required to produce this special examination. The contrast agent used is water-soluble, tri-iodinated compound. A commonly used agent is meglumine diatrizoate and sodium diatrizoate (RenoCal–76 distributed by Bracco Diagnostics, Princeton, NJ but many agents with high iodine concentration can be used). Contrast agents with 50-76% concentrations are utilized in equine fistulography because the soft tissue thickness is often great. An assortment of delivery agents is recommended for this procedure including teat cannulas, plastic intravenous catheters, and Foley catheters. A 4-inch, 10 or 12-gauge teat cannula is the preferred delivery agent used in our practice. An assortment of Foley catheter sizes is desirable, but the recommended size for common use in equine practice is a 30-French with a 35-cc inflatable cuff.

The opening of a draining tract should be marked using a BB or other small dense marker taped to the skin at the opening of the draining lesion prior to producing the radiographs (Figures 3-3A, B, C). If the relationship between a chronic periosteal reaction and a fistulous tract is unknown, fistulography is indicated to establish the relationship (Figure 3-3D). Survey radiographs must be taken and interpreted for signs of cellulitis prior to insertion of a catheter. Clipping the hair coat and cleaning the region is advised to aid in reducing artifacts. It is recommended that as aseptic a technique as possible be used. Insert the sterile catheter into the draining tract, carefully probing the tract to get as deep into the lesion as possible. When the tract opening is large, the use of a Foley catheter is recommended. The balloon on the Foley catheter should be inflated with sterile water to provide a soft tissue-equivalent background density. The volume of contrast agent varies greatly according to the tract size, depth, and communicating regions. For a simple tract on the distal limb, 10-20 cc of contrast is usually sufficient. Inject the contrast agent in the area and continue to do so as the catheter is slowly retracted. Digital pressure should be applied at the tract opening and an absorbing material should be used to minimize outflow of the agent onto the skin. Radiographs are made using at least two orthogonal projections that profile the area. A second examination should be done *approximately 10-15 minutes* after the first to help identify or confirm radiolucent foreign bodies. When multiple draining tracts are present, each should be injected if contrast does not flow out following prior injections (Figure 3-4). If there is a question of the tract communicating with a joint space, it may be easier to do an aseptic intra-articular contrast injection of the joint. The joint should be injected at a site away from the tract. The increased intra-articular pressure created by the contrast injection should permit the communication between the joint space and draining tract to be identified if one exists (Figure 3-5).

Interpretation of the fistulogram should be directed at determining the cause of the draining tract, direction and extent of the tract, and communication of the tract with a tendon sheath, joint space, or bursa. The cause of the tract may be a foreign body, osteomyelitis with or without seques-tration, or chronic infection. The most difficult cause to identify is a lucent foreign body. The radiographic signs of a radiolucent foreign body are a filling defect in the contrast and straight, sharp margination of the defect (Figure 3-6). The foreign body often can be identified more easily on the 10 to 15-minute follow-up radiographs because the contrast volume is reduced and the foreign body may be highlighted by a thin coat of contrast material.

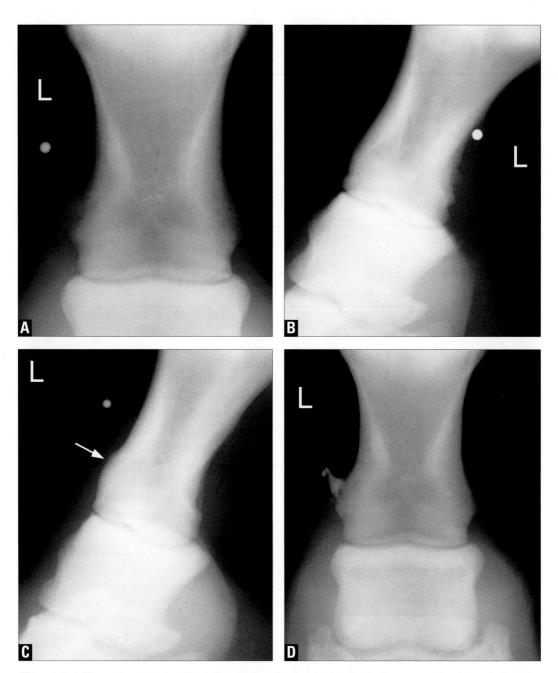

Figure 3-3. *A BB was taped to the skin at the opening of a draining tract prior to exposure for determination of a relationship between the opening of a draining lesion and the underlying bone (**A**). The medial (**B**) and lateral oblique (**C**) views revealed the chronic periosteal reaction was located at the lateral and palmarolateral regions of the distal P-1 with only a minor degree being on the dorsolateral region (arrow). Note the variation in sizes of the BB resulting from magnification. Fistulography revealed the fistulous tract communicated with the area of chronic periosteal reaction (**D**).*

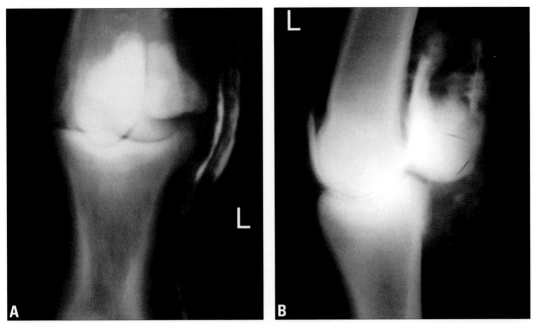

Figure 3-4. Multiple draining tracts require each be injected unless the injection of one results in contrast outflow from all openings. Injection of a palmar fetlock tract resulted in contrast identified within a tendon sheath (*A*). The second tract was injected and communication with the fetlock joint space was established by contrast being identified dorsally and in the palmar pouches (*B*).

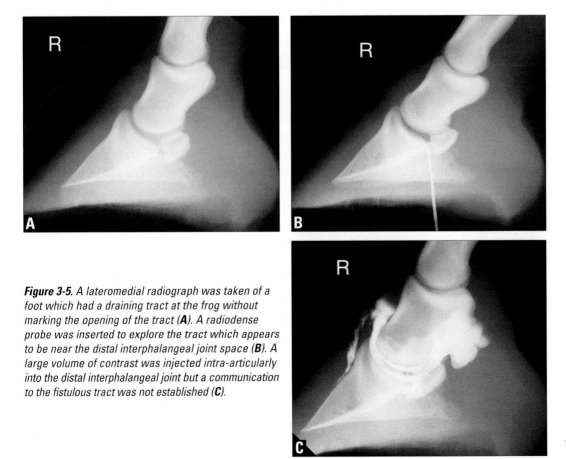

Figure 3-5. A lateromedial radiograph was taken of a foot which had a draining tract at the frog without marking the opening of the tract (*A*). A radiodense probe was inserted to explore the tract which appears to be near the distal interphalangeal joint space (*B*). A large volume of contrast was injected intra-articularly into the distal interphalangeal joint but a communication to the fistulous tract was not established (*C*).

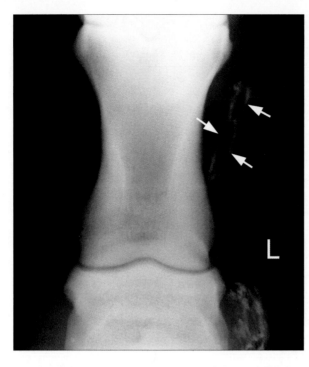

Figure 3-6. *Fistulography is extremely valuable for diagnosing a lucent foreign body. The radiographic signs of a lucent foreign body are a filling defect in the contrast (compare to a tract without a filling defect [Figure 3-3D]) and straight, sharp margination of this defect (arrows). This radiographic view was taken 10-15 minutes following the contrast injection resulting in the foreign body (wood) being highlighted by the thin coat of contrast. The referring AEPs failed to identify this foreign body on the excellent quality fistulogram they produced resulting in re-evaluation ten weeks later (see Figure 3-2).*

In summary, survey radiographs must be taken before doing fistulography. Fistulography is a special radiographic examination. A separate examination fee should be charged that is justified by one's expertise for knowing when fistulography is indicated, how to perform the procedure, and the interpretation of the radiographs.

II. Radiographic Interpretation of Bone Infection

Introduction

Radiographic interpretation of infection of bone in the horse must be based on the age of the horse and the morphology of bone involved with this disease process. The recommended format for evaluating radiographic findings in the horse and the one utilized in this chapter is:

- Adult Horse: Osteomyelitis of a bone with a distinct cortex of compact bone and a well-defined periosteum.
- Adult Horse: Osteomyelitis of a bone without both a distinct cortex of compact bone and a well-defined periosteum.
- Immature Horse: Hematogenous osteomyelitis

1. Adult Horse: Osteomyelitis of a bone with a distinct cortex of compact bone and a well-defined periosteum

Bone infection in the adult horse is usually limited to one area and it is often commonly associated with a penetrating wound, degloving injury, or a contaminated fracture. Hematogenous osteomyelitis is uncommon in the adult horse. An infection produces inflammation that can involve the periosteum, cortex or the medullary cavity. The radiographic conclusion is limited in precision for diagnosing infection of the bone. The pathologist can describe the morphologic changes as a periosteitis, osteitis, or osteomyelitis. One cannot be this specific interpreting radiographs so when a destructive-productive lesion is identified involving the periosteum, cortex, or medullary cavity, it is concluded to be an osteomyelitis. Therefore, osteomyelitis is a common radiographic conclusion in the horse. The exception occurs when there is a periosteal bony response without evidence of cortical and medullary involvement in a patient with clinical signs of a related soft tissue infection. The radiographic conclusion for a patient with these conditions is a periosteitis caused by induction.

Radiographic signs evaluated in a patient suspected to have osteomyelitis are:
- **Extracapsular soft tissue swelling**
- **Irregularity to the surface contour of the STS**
- **Abnormal tissue density within the E-STS, i.e., decreased (gas) or increased (foreign body or debris)**
- **Presence of productive, destructive, or a combination productive–destructive bony change.**

These four findings vary in degree and presence depending on the duration of the osteomyelitis. A clinical example will demonstrate the application of these diagnostic signs during the earlier, middle, and later phases of an osteomyelitis following a large laceration to the dorsum of the first phalanx.

A. Earlier Phase of Osteomyelitis
Horses with clinical signs of <u>osteomyelitis less than 7-10 days</u> are generally expected to have the following radiographic signs:
- **Prominent E-STS including defects when associated with a laceration or degloving injury (Figure 3-7).**
- **If the swelling is secondary to a skin laceration or penetration:**
  - **Irregular surface contour to the E-STS**
  - **Decreased density in STS secondary to gas or a tissue defect**
  - **Increased density in the STS secondary to foreign body or debris**
  - **Shallow lucent defect(s) in the cortical surface secondary to direct trauma**
- **No evidence of a fracture. Productive bony changes are usually not seen in less than 7 days.**

In fact, the findings during the acute phase are essentially those of cellulitis without bony reactive changes.

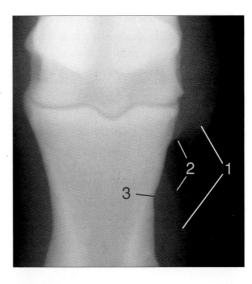

Figure 3-7. Radiographic signs seen with the early phase of osteomyelitis in the adult horse associated with a skin laceration include prominent E-STS with an irregular surface contour (1), decreased density in the STS secondary to gas accumulation (2), and irregular cortical surface secondary to direct traumatic injury (3). Foreign body, debris, and a fracture are not seen.

B. Middle Phase of Osteomyelitis
Most horses presented for radiographic examination at our hospital with a clinical diagnosis of osteomyelitis have a duration of the condition ranging <u>from 7-10 days to a few weeks.</u> The radiographic findings seen in the adult horse in this time interval are modifications of those seen in the earlier phase (Figure 3-8).

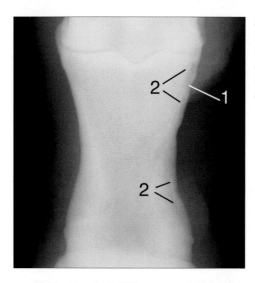

Figure 3-8. The radiographic signs seen in Figure 3-7 two weeks later included persistent E-STS with irregular surface contour and cortical bone destruction at the surface (1) and as linear lucencies running parallel to bone surface (2). Periosteal bony production and a distinct sequestration are not identified.

- Reduction in E-STS may or may not be seen.
- More irregular contour to the surface of the E-STS
- Cortical bone destruction first seen as a linear lucency at the surface or within the cortex running parallel to the bony surface.
- A dense, sharply marginated osseous body (sequestrum) may be seen in the cortex.
- Periosteal bony production or periosteal new bone growth (PNBG) that has an irregular appearance to its surface may be visualized at the bony surface. If there is an area of sequestration, the PNBG will be seen surrounding it.

C. Later Phase of Osteomyelitis

The radiographic signs expected in an adult horse with <u>osteomyelitis of more than a month</u> are modifications of those described for the earlier and middle phases.
- More focal E-STS may or may not be seen.
- Contour of skin surface may be either smoother (if healing has occurred) or irregular (if granulation tissue has overgrown the area).
- Cortical bone destruction may have progressed and a dense, sharply marginated osseous body or bodies may be seen separated from the parent bone (Figure 3-9). This body often has a lucent zone surrounding and highlighting it.

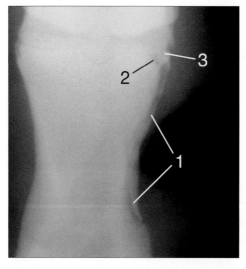

Figure 3-9. The radiographic signs seen in Figure 3-7 have progressed at four weeks and include additional cortical bone destruction with osseous bodies (1) separating from the body of P-1 and the chronic osteomyelitis has extended into the fetlock joint (2) resulting in infectious arthritis and a pathological fracture (3). As a result of the extensiveness of the lateral cortical involvement (sequestration) a periosteal reaction is minimal being seen distal to the sequestra.

- **The parent bone has evidence of a greater degree of bony productive response resulting in more density to the area adjacent to the origin of the separated bony fragment (involucrum).**
- **Extensive PNBG. This periosteal response tends to be more extensive in area and more uniform in density.**
- **Occasionally the chronic osteomyelitis may extend into a joint (see Figure 3-9).**

A knowledge of the structural changes seen radiographically in the horse with osteomyelitis requires an understanding of the related pathology of a bone infection. The pathology can be correlated to the clinical and radiographic signs of an osteomyelitis with sequestration.

	Pathology	Radiographic Signs	Clinical Signs
Infection of Bone	hyperemia + edema + exudation		pain
	spreads through the haversian and Volkmann canals		
	septic emboli compromise circulation		
	bone necrosis and separation at interface between viable and non-viable bone	sequestrum	
	fluid from breakdown products increased and elevates the periosteum	lucent zone surrounding sequestrum and periosteal reaction	
	rupture of periosteum	cloaca	
	fluid dissects tissues	sinus tract	
	discharge at the skin surface		fistula

A sequestrum is defined as a dead piece of bone. When associated with a clinical problem in the horse the sequestrum is usually infected.

Bones without a significant amount of overlying soft tissue protection are more susceptible to osteomyelitis with sequestration from degloving injuries and open wounds. These bones in the horse include the dorsum of the first and second phalanges, third metacarpus/metatarsus, distodorsal radius and tibia. Injury can produce a loss of periosteal blood supply to the dorsum of these bones. The outer cortex (~1/3) is without blood supply while the remaining cortex (~2/3) has blood supply from the endosteal side.

Osteolysis occurs at junction between avascular and vascular bone producing a linear lucent area in the dorsal cortex. This linear lucency often runs parallel to the surface of the bone, and it is the first bony radiographic sign commonly seen usually occurring at approximately 10-14 days. Dorsal to this linear lucency the bone is devoid of the periosteal blood supply and will form a sequestrum.

The lucent zone contains purulent material and granulation tissue. The bone in this area with blood supply will become sclerotic with time as it "walls-off" the disease process producing the involucrum. The sequestrum appears radiographically to be sharply marginated and more dense than the bone where it originated (Figure 3-10). This is explained by the fact it is a dead piece of bone having the density of the original bone, and the adjacent bone is reduced in density by the initial hyperemia created by the blood flow from the medullary side and the exudate creating resorption. Radiographic evidence of periosteal new bone production is soon seen surrounding the margins of the lesion resulting from the periosteum with blood supply being stimulated by the disease process.

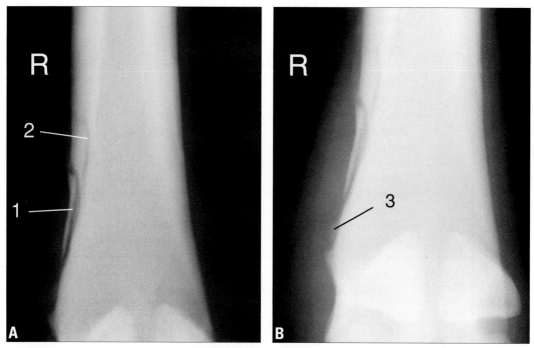

Figure 3-10. A sharply marginated, dense bony fragment (1) indicative of a sequestrum is seen at the surface of the distolateral cortex of the right MTIII *(A)*. Another larger bony body (2) is seen proximal to the more apparent dense body (1) because of the linear lucency which represents the junction between avascular and vascular bone. A slightly obliqued view *(B)* at a reduced exposure time (t=x/2) permits the E-STS and early periosteal reaction to be seen distally (3).

2. Adult Horse: Osteomyelitis of a bone with an indistinct cortex of compact bone and a poorly-defined periosteum

The radiographic features and signs of osteomyelitis in the adult horse previously described are seen in bones with a distinct cortex of compact bone and a well-defined periosteum. The radiographic signs in some bones without a distinct cortex of compact bone and complete periosteum vary. The two best examples of such bones in the horse are the abaxial part of the proximal sesamoid bones and the third phalanx.

A comparison of the radiographic signs seen in <u>the proximal sesamoid bones and third phalanx</u> to those described for compact cortical bone are:

- **A defined E-STS associated with the bony changes is more difficult to identify especially involving P3.**
- **The bony lesion is primarily a destructive change (Figure 3-11).**
- **Any productive change is identified as a "walling-off" attempt with a minor degree or absence of periosteal response.**
- **A sequestrum is uncommonly seen and when identified tends to be very small.**

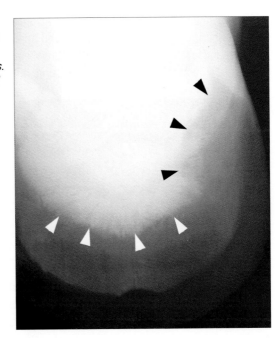

Figure 3-11. Osteomyelitis of the third phalanx is primarily seen radiographically as a destructive lesion (black arrowheads) where the bone appears to "melt away" when seen on serial radiographic examinations. The abnormal contour to P-3 at the medial and lateral toe regions (white arrowheads) are secondary to pathological fractures.

Management of Osteomyelitis with Sequestration

Surgery and curettage are required to successfully treat osteomyelitis with sequestration. The involucrum should be curetted until the surface blood supply has been established that will permit healing of the lesion. Antibiotic therapy is usually unnecessary if the sequestrum and remaining necrotic tissues are completely debrided.

It is important that the radiographic examination permits the complications of an osteomyelitis to be evaluated. Important complications include a pathological fracture, extension of the bone infection into a joint or growth plate, or a chronic osteomyelitis. A chronic osteomyelitis resulting in periodic drainage can present a difficult clinical management problem.

Such a clinical dilemma results from the radiographic examination that reveals a bony cavitary lesion typical of sequestration, but a sequestrum cannot be seen radiographically. A sequestrum cannot be identified even though the exposure technique may be reduced and additional radiographs are taken with different angulation and degrees of obliquity. It is possible that the sequestrum has been "flushed" from the cavitary lesion by drainage from the site of the lesion or the sequestrum may be so small it cannot be seen radiographically. The clinical signs must be the governing factor in managing this situation. If there is no discharge associated with the area, a conservative treatment approach is recommended. If a discharge recurs, surgery with curettage of the bony cavitary lesion is indicated.

3. Immature Horse: Hematogenous Osteomyelitis

The diagnosis of a hematogenous bone infection is usually made on the clinical history and signs. The history of a foal not getting colostrum within the first 12-18 hours of life is commonly associated with a hematogenous infection. The clinical signs of fever, lameness, swelling near joints, and pain to palpation further support the clinical diagnosis. The primary objectives of the radiographic examination are to determine where the bony changes are located and the extent of any bony changes. Hematogenous infections often begin as an infectious synovitis that extends into the joint then bone. A hematogenous osteomyelitis may be epiphyseal, metaphyseal, or diaphyseal as well as being monostotic or polyostotic. In addition, a monostotic involvement may occur as single or multiple lesions. The radiographic evaluation of a metaphyseal lesion must include a careful analysis of the physis and adjacent epiphysis (Figure 3-12). When the metaphyseal lesion extends across the physis and into the epiphysis, the growth potential of the area will be compromised because the stem cells of the physis lose blood supply.

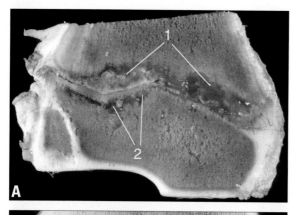

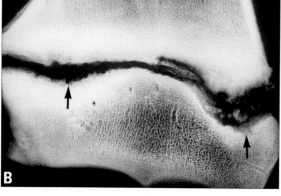

Figure 3-12. Hematogenous osteomyelitis in the foal commonly begins in the metaphyseal side (1) of the growth center, but it may extend across the physis (2) into the epiphysis **(A)**. This results in a compromised blood supply to the stem cells of the physis and loss of growth potential. The radiographic evaluation **(B)** must include a careful analysis for destruction (irregularity) on the epiphyseal side of the growth plate (arrows).

The radiographic signs of a hematogenous osteomyelitis are:
- **Extracapsular STS when the bony changes do not involve the subchondral bone of a joint.**
- **Focal or regional destructive bony lesion(s) when metaphyseal or epiphyseal in location.**
- **Initially the destructive metaphyseal bony lesion tends to have a rounded appearance which changes in shape and size with duration. This shape and enlargement results as the disease process extends abaxially, axially, and distally into the metaphysis.**
- **Loss of the subchondral plate for the physis indicates extension into the epiphysis and loss of blood supply to the stem cells of the growth plate.**

Interpretation of early radiographic signs may be difficult in the foal because signs of bone destruction may be subtle, soft tissue swelling compromises assessment of bony detail, and the veterinarian's knowledge of normal variation in radiographic appearances of growth plates and epiphyses with age, sex, and breed may be marginal. These factors can lead to confusion and inaccurate radiographic conclusions and impressions.

The solution to this common problem for the equine practitioner is a comparison radiographic examination of the same anatomical area of the opposite limb. **This comparison technique should be part of the routine examination procedure for foals with potential bone, joint, and growth plate disorders**. Interpretation by having comparison radiographs will usually eliminate the problems of subtle destructive change and a lack of knowledge for normality variations related to age, sex, and breed. However, one must always be aware that hematogenous osteomyelitis can be polyostotic so integrate the clinical examination findings into your interpretation. Furthermore, when changes are seen bilaterally, there is nearly always a variation in the degree of radiographic signs seen when comparing the anatomical area of interest.

III. Radiographic Interpretation of Joint Disease

Radiographic evaluation of joints is a very common procedure for the equine practitioner. There are two clinical diagnoses responsible for most radiographic examination of joint. The less common of the two is infectious arthritis (IA) and the much more common is secondary joint disease (SJD). SJD is the preferred term to degenerative joint disease because SJD is more inclusive and does not identify a specific etiology such as degeneration. In fact, joint disease resulting from conformation weaknesses and acute traumatic events frequently produces joint disease in the horse that should be classified as SJD rather than a true degenerative disorder. The end stage of IA following successful treatment also produces radiographic signs compatible with a diagnosis of SJD.

1. Infectious Arthritis

Infectious arthritis is a very serious clinical disorder, and it is important to understand the role of radiology in patients suspected to have IA. This role can be summarized as "Don't waste a lot of time on radiology in the patient suspected to have acute joint infection." Take a radiographic examination to establish a baseline reference point and exclude fractures and subchondral lytic lesions, then do arthrocentesis because IA is a clinical diagnosis.

The radiographic interpretation of acute IA is based on a knowledge of how the joint was infected. There are three major mechanisms leading to joint infection:
- Hematogenous synovitis with extension into a joint space.
- Osteomyelitis of the subchondral bone with extension into a joint.
- Iatrogenic introduction.

A. Acute IA

Acute IA commonly occurs in foals. The IA develops from synovitis which spreads into the joint space. **The radiographic signs in <u>acute IA</u> are:**
- **Intracapsular STS (I-STS).**
- **Subchondral bone assessment for fracture lines or osteolytic lesion(s) compatible with osteomyelitis.**
- **Lucency within the joint capsule compatible with intracapsular gas.**
- **Increased width to joint space secondary to increased joint fluid pressure and non-weight bearing when the radiographs were taken (remember a three-legged lameness is the main clinical sign in these patients).**
- **Periarticular productive changes are not seen in the acute phase.**

B. Subacute IA

An infection of a joint for <u>more than seven days</u> is considered subacute. **The radiographic signs are:**
- **I-STS and E-STS.**
- **Increased lucency in the subchondral bone commonly producing an abnormal contour.**
- **Widening of the joint space if the horse is non-weight bearing at the time of radiography. If weight-bearing, there is an overall narrowing of the joint space. The subchondral bony lucency can produce focal areas of joint space widening within the overall narrowed joint space.**
- **Low density, small periarticular osteophytes around the joint margins.**
- **Younger horses will have primarily destructive marginal change. Older horses tend to have more productive marginal changes at the joint.**

C. Chronic IA

<u>Chronic IA</u> represents an unsuccessfully treated acute or subacute IA. The radiographic signs are also an extension of those seen in the earlier phases of the disease process but they are of a greater degree.
- **Persistent STS**
- **Subchondral lucencies produce an irregular contour to the articular surface**
- **Sclerosis develops surrounding the subchondral lucencies**
- **Loss of the joint space**
- **Extensive periarticular remodeling change resulting in an increased size to the joint space**

The end-point of an unsuccessfully treated IA can be fusion or ankylosis of the joint. The radiographic signs of ankylosis are loss of the lucent joint space with periarticular and periosteal productive changes at the margins of the articulation. Ankylosis in the horse tends to occur as an end-stage joint change at the carpometacarpal, tarsometatarsal, distal intertarsal, and proximal interphalangeal joints. High motion joints are more likely to become larger secondary to periarticular and periosteal productive changes with reduced range of motion. However, radiographic signs of ankylosis are less likely in the high motion joint.

2. Secondary Joint Disease

The expected end stage for both a successfully treated osteomyelitis that extended into a joint and IA is SJD, but SJD in the horse more commonly results from trauma. Horses are subjected to hard work on a daily basis resulting in trauma to joints. This trauma may be severe producing an acute injury, e.g., fracture, but more commonly it produces repetitive micro-trauma to equine joints that is subclinical for a long period of time. The degree of trauma and the range of joint motion influences the radiographic signs of SJD. Other factors including conformational abnormalities, developmental disorders, and damage to supporting structures of a joint also contribute to the severity of the radiographic findings associated with traumatic SJD. The severity of radiographic signs with an infectious SJD is dependent on the severity and duration of the infection and the effectiveness of treatment.

It is important to emphasize that a direct correlation between the degree of radiographic signs and the severity of clinical signs in traumatic SJD <u>cannot</u> be made for the horse. Furthermore, the degree of clinical signs cannot negate the significance of radiographic findings of SJD seen during purchase examinations. An excellent example to emphasize this important point is found in canine hip dysplasia. A young German Shepherd dog is presented to you for a pelvic radiographic examination leading to certification for an absence of hip dysplasia. The owner swears this dog has never been lame in its life and has been worked hard. Your interpretation of the dog's radiographs determines there are radiographic signs of bilateral shallow acetabula, a moderate degree of subluxation of the coxofemoral joints and extensive periarticular remodeling changes of the femoral necks. These morphologic changes document hip dysplasia with SJD even though clinical signs are not evident.

The major radiographic signs of SJD are:
- **Intracapsular joint capsule distention.**
- **Perarticular remodeling changes.**
- **Narrowing of the joint space.**
- **Subchondral sclerosis.**
- **Periosteal productive changes in more chronic conditions.**
- **Periarticular and subchrondral cystic lucencies in more chronic conditions especially with infectious SJD.**

The intracapsular distension is secondary to increased fluid resulting from a synovitis. The periarticular remodeling change is productive resulting in periarticular osteophytes formation and development as the duration of the process becomes longer. These osteophytes are commonly seen best on obliqued radiographs of the joint (Figure 3-13). At the fetlock the osteophytes tend to be seen first at the dorsum of proximal P-1 and later at the dorsum of distal MC3. It is expected to see this sequence of osteophyte development occur and is a result of direct contact associated with joint movement. This effect is referred to as a "kissing" lesion. The cartilage becomes thinner with wear from continued stress and poor nutrition from the diluted synovial fluid resulting in the subchondral bone being closer together. The subchondral bone impacting without the buffering influence of the articular cartilage leads to subchondral sclerosis. Periosteal productive change around the joint is seen with longer duration and is attributed to a greater range of motion

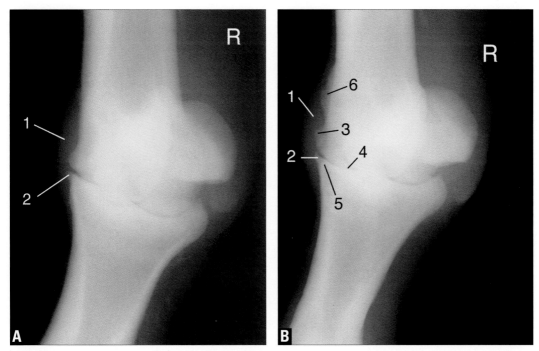

Figure 3-13. *The radiographic signs of secondary joint disease (SJD) are commonly seen at the fetlock joint and in the earlier stages **(A)** include: I-STS (1) and small periarticular remodeling change (2) at the dorsum of proximal P-1. Progression of SJD **(B)** is characterized by persistence of intracapsular joint capsule distention (1), enlargement of the periarticular osteophytes on dorsoproximal P-1 (2) and development on dorsodistal MCIII (3), narrowing of the width of the joint space (4), development of subchondral sclerosis best seen on the dorsoproximal P-1 (5), and periosteal productive changes at the dorsodistal MCIII (6).*

producing more damage to the attachment of the fibrous part of the joint capsule. Periarticular and subchondral lucencies can be identified in certain equine joints with chronic SJD.

Periarticular cystic lucencies are frequently seen on the palmar aspect of the proximal interphalangeal joint and the palmarodistal third metacarpus. Subchondral lucencies are commonly seen at the distal intertarsal joint with chronic secondary joint disease. In fact, these subchondral lucencies in any other joint of the horse would be compatible with an infectious arthritis.

NOTES

NOTES

NOTES

NOTES

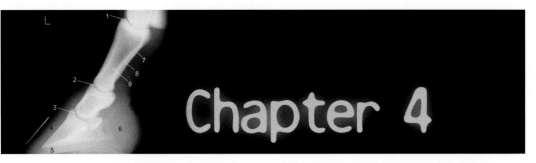

Chapter 4

Radiography of the Distal Extremity

I. Introduction

II. Preparation of the Foot

III. Production Items for the Distal Extremity Examination (DEE)

IV. Positioning the Foot to Examine A Horse with Foot Lameness

V. Technique Settings for the DEE

VI. Conclusions

I. Introduction

The three components needed for an accurate radiographic interpretation of the DEE are:
- Diagnostic quality radiographs
- An adequate number of radiographic projections per examination
- Basic knowledge of radiographic findings seen with the DEE

This chapter deals with the first two of these components and the third is dealt with in Chapter 5.

Diagnostic quality radiographs were discussed in general in Chapter 1. There is additional information relative to the DEE that must be presented and emphasized. Diagnostic quality radiographs of the distal extremity are a function of foot preparation, positioning, and production.

II. Preparation of the Foot

Lack of preparation of the equine foot is a major cause of non-diagnostic radiographs. Proper foot preparation must be utilized to eliminate artifacts. Preparation includes:
- Removal of the shoe
- Cleaning of the foot to remove dirt and debris
- Elimination of excessive horny tissue
- Packing the sulci of the frog with a soft tissue equivalent material to eliminate gas artifacts (Figure 4-1)

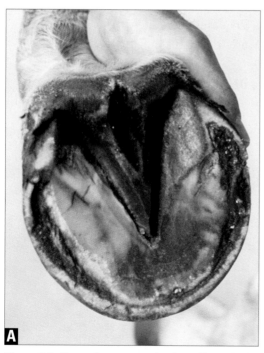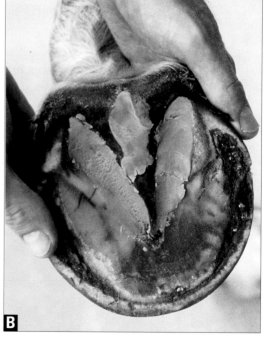

Figure 4-1. *Proper foot preparation for radiography is an essential part of the DEE. The shoe has been removed, the foot scrubbed to remove debris (**A**), and the sulci have been packed (**B**).*

The items required by the AEP for proper foot preparation are:
- Shoe removal equipment
- Hoof knife, pick, and rasp
- Scrub brush
- Packing material
- 2' x 2' heavy canvas

Foot preparation items must be utilized to eliminate artifacts. Many distal extremity examinations cannot be completely or correctly interpreted because of inadequate foot preparation. Cleaning the foot carefully and packing the sole and sulci of the frog are required to make the soft tissues uniform in density and eliminate artifacts. Often veterinarians complain that shoe removal and foot preparation including scrubbing the hoof wall require too much time and effort. A solution to this problem has been to have the veterinarian advise owners that they can save the value of one-half to one hour of the veterinarian's time if they will have the shoe removed from the lame foot, the foot scrubbed clean, and then wrapped in a watertight, heavy plastic bag before your arrival.

The packing material utilized must be soft-tissue equivalent in density. Do not pack the foot beyond the apex of the frog to avoid artifacts at the solar margin of PIII in the toe region. A commercial modeling compound is recommended because of its density, availability, and inexpensiveness (Play-Doh, Hasbro, Inc., Pawtucket, RI).

A 2' x 2' heavy canvas is put on the ground for the horse to stand upon after foot preparation and packing. This eliminates artifacts produced by debris accumulating in the packing material. This canvas also provides a wrapping material for storage of the foot preparation items when not in use.

III. Production Items for the DEE

There are items needed for the DEE that permit proper positioning, identification, and radiation safety. These items with an estimated cost in 2004 dollars are:

1. Positioning items
Slotted wooden block ($45)
Tunnel cassette holder ($65)
Aluminum frame 8"x10" cassette holder with a 12" arm ($115)
Tripod x-ray stand ($300)

A slotted wooden block is needed for exposure of the lateromedial (LM) and dorso 45° proximal-palmarodistal oblique (45°DP) projections. A tunnel cassette holder is needed for both dorso 65° proximal-palmarodistal oblique projections and the extended palmaro 50° proximal-palmarodistal oblique projection. It is critical that the horse not be allowed to stand upon the unprotected cassette because replacement of damaged cassettes is expensive as was discussed in Chapter 2.

The aluminum frame cassette holders for 8"x10" cassettes can be purchased with detachable 12" and 30" arms. Most AEP utilize the 12" arm because it is more efficiently used and can provide adequate protection. The cassette holder should be constructed with a handle that is adjustable for positioning.

2. Identification items

Lead markers: Right/left/fore/hind (100 markers approximately $100)
Dorsal hoof wall identification: wire, solder or barium paste (minimal expense)

Proper radiographic identification is a requirement to avoid legal and medical controversies. Identification of the extremity before exposure must be done because the limb and laterality cannot be accurately determined from anatomical features of the distal extremity on the radiographs. Patient information should be incorporated into the radiograph prior to film processing.

3. Radiation safety items

Dosimetry: Start-up fees plus two badges with quarterly readings approximately $158 per annum
Protective lead aprons ($120 each) and gloves ($129 per pair) that have 0.5 mm lead quivalence.

Radiation safety items listed are a requirement! They are listed here even though they are used for radiographic examinations in general. It must be emphasized that the veterinarian is responsible for the radiation safety associated with producing the radiographic examination.

IV. Positioning the Foot to Examine a Horse with Foot Lameness

1. How Many Projections Should be Taken?

The answer to this question is related to the objective of the radiographic examination. If a laminitis evaluation is the objective, two views are required. Otherwise, a routine DEE consisting of five views should be taken. If there is doubt concerning which examination will be more diagnostic, perform the routine DEE because it will permit a more complete evaluation of the foot.

The examination for laminitis consists of a lateromedial (LM) and a dorsopalmar projection for the third phalanx or 65°DP-P3. The descriptive terminology for this projection is dorso 65°proximal-palmarodistal oblique*.

2. The Views for the Routine DEE

A routine distal extremity examination allows radiographic evaluation of the phalanges, interphalangeal joints, navicular bone, and hoof wall. Five radiographic projections are needed for a routine examination to evaluate the above anatomical areas.

1. Lateromedial Projection (LM)
A. TECHNIQUE

A small wire should be taped on the dorsal aspect of the hoof to delineate the surface of the dorsal hoof wall, and the foot should be placed on a positioning block. Identification markers should be taped on the cassette in front of the foot. To prevent obliquity, one of the most common causes of poor quality for this projection, line up the beam with the bulbs of the heel superimposed. The beam should be directed parallel to the ground with the x-ray beam centered at the coronary band midway between the dorsal and palmar surfaces (Figure 4-2).

* Descriptive terminology is explained in detail in Chapter 5 under Section II-2-B.

B. COMMON PROBLEMS

1. Obliquity
2. Not marking the dorsal hoof wall surface
3. Excessive collimation resulting in loss of the toe region of P3

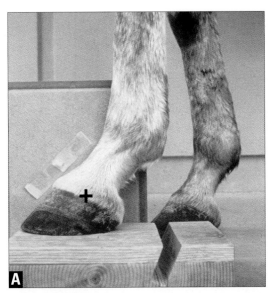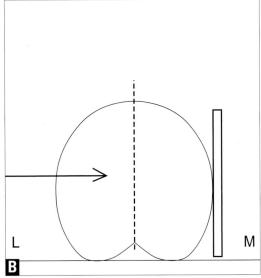

Figure 4-2. The LM projection is exposed with the foot on a positioning block *(A)*, the central x-ray beam perpendicular and centered (X) at the coronary band midway between the dorsal and palmar surfaces, and the bulbs of the heels superimposed *(B)* to prevent obliquity.

C. ANATOMICAL AREAS EVALUATED

The LM radiograph permits the dorsal and palmar surfaces of the phalanges and interphalangeal joints to be highlighted (Figure 4-3). The dorsal hoof wall thickness, the soft tissues of the solar and heel regions, the proximal and distal borders of the navicular bone, and the contour of the flexor cortex of the navicular bone can also be evaluated. Evaluation of the thickness of the dorsal hoof wall is enhanced by placing a radiodense wire or barium paste on the dorsal surface. This must be done if the radiograph is overexposed which does not permit the dorsal surface of the hoof wall to be clearly visualized. The thickness of the dorsal

Figure 4-3. The LM view permits optimum evaluation of the dorsal and palmar (plantar) aspects of the following anatomical areas:
• Periarticular and subchondral regions of the metacarpophalangeal (1), proximal interphalangeal (2) and distal interphalangeal (3) joints.
• The dorsal hoof wall (4), solar (5), and heel (6) regions.
• Periosteal (7), cortical (8), and medullary (9) regions of the distal third metacarpus, first, second, and third phalanges and navicular bone.

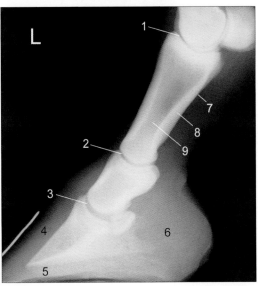

hoof wall will range from 15-18 mm for most breeds of horses (see Chapter 6 for details of the measuring technique and interpretation).

2. Dorso 45°Proximal-Palmarodistal Oblique (45°DP)
A. TECHNIQUE
The 45°DP is produced with the limb fully weight-bearing and the foot on the positioning block with the cassette behind the foot in the slotted groove of the block. The opposite limb is elevated when needed to make the horse fully weight bearing. The x-ray beam is directed from the dorsoproximal to palmarodistal perpendicular to the pastern which is approximately 45° to the ground. The beam is centered at midline one to two inches above the coronary band (at the level of the proximal interphalangeal joint), and collimated to include the metacarpophalangeal joint and P3. Identifying markers are placed on the cassette at the lateral aspect within the collimated area to identify the limb (Figure 4-4).

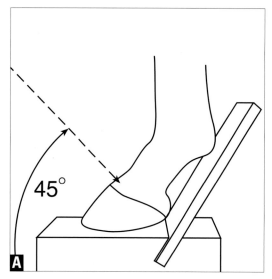

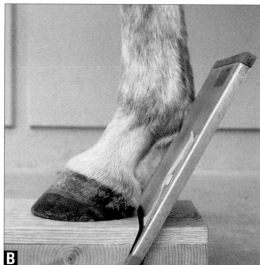

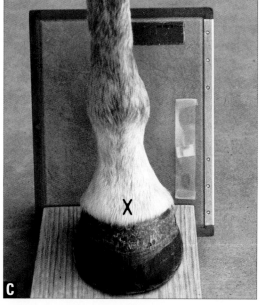

Figure 4-4. *The 45°DP projection is exposed with the cassette in the slot of the positioning block using an x-ray beam directed from the dorso45°proximal to the palmarodistal direction **(A, B)**. The beam is centered (X) approximately one inch proximal to the coronary band at midline **(C)**.*

B. COMMON PROBLEMS

1. Substituting the D0°Pr-PaDiO for the 45°DP
2. Not identifying the lateral aspect of the foot
3. Not including the metacarpophalangeal joint
4. Placing the cassette blocker over the images of the navicular bone and third phalanx

C. ANATOMICAL REGIONS EVALUATED

The 45°DP projection permits interpretation of the proximal border and body of the navicular bone, medial and lateral surfaces of the phalanges and collateral cartilages, and the metacarpophalangeal and interphalangeal joints (Figure 4-5). These joints should be evaluated for width, marginal productive changes, and subchondral bony density abnormalities. As a rule of thumb, the joint space widths of the proximal interphalangeal joint should be 50% and the metacarpophalangeal 40% of the width of the distal interphalangeal joint.

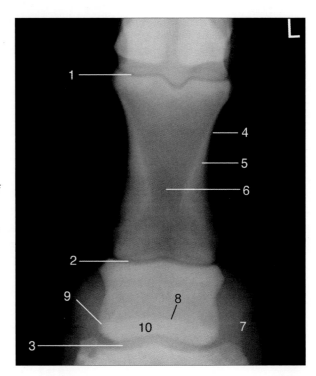

Figure 4-5. The 45°DP view permits optimum evaluation of the medial and lateral aspects of the following anatomical areas:
• Periarticular and subchondral regions and joint space width of the metacarpophalangeal (1), proximal interphalangeal (2) and distal interphalangeal (3) joints.
• Periosteal (4), cortical (5), and medullary (6) regions of the distal third metacarpus, first, second, and third phalanges.
• The heel and collateral cartilage regions (7).
• Navicular bone: The proximal border (8), extremities (9), and proximal two-thirds of the body (10).

3. Dorso 65°Proximal-Palmarodistal Oblique of P3 (65°DP-P3)

A. TECHNIQUE

The foot is centered on the cassette tunnel containing the cassette with the toe near the front edge and identification markers on the lateral aspect of the foot. The x-ray unit is elevated 65° and the exposure is made from the dorsoproximal to palmarodistal direction. The beam is centered on midline at the coronary band and the entirety of P3 including the toe should be in the field of exposure (Figure 4-6).

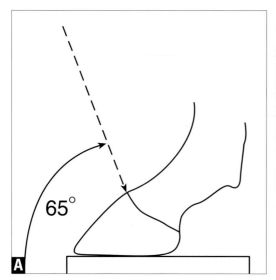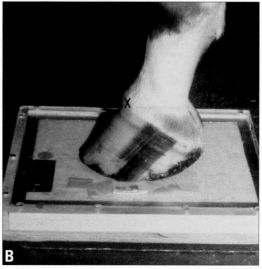

Figure 4-6. *The positioning for the dorso65°proximal-palmarodistal oblique view for the third phalanx (65°DP-P3) is illustrated **(A)** and placement of the foot on the cassette tunnel is shown **(B)**. The central x-ray beam is centered at the coronary band and a limb identification marker is seen near the lateral quarter, as it should be on all views taken in the dorsopalmar direction.*

B. COMMON PROBLEMS

1. Overexposure of the solar margin of P3
2. Obliquity from the DP plane
3. Positioning so the toe region of P3 is not seen on the radiograph

C. ANATOMICAL AREAS EVALUATED

The 65°DP-P3 is taken primarily to evaluate the horny wall, solar margin, and the body of P3 (Figure 4-7). Many AEP overexpose this view so the solar margin cannot be evaluated for contour abnormalities including irregularities, defects, and fractures. It is recommended that most AEP reduce their exposure time by a factor of two or four to increase the diagnostic quality of the 65°DP-P3 (see Figure 9, Chapter 6).

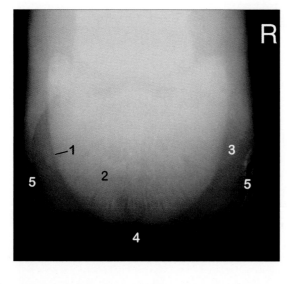

Figure 4-7. *The 65°DP-P3 view permits optimum evaluation of the following anatomical areas:*
* *Solar margin (1)*
* *Distal body of P3 (2)*
* *Hoof wall in the quarter (3) and toe (4) regions*
* *Note the artifacts in the hoof wall both medially and laterally associated with debris in the nail tracks (5).*

4. Dorso 65°Proximal-Palmarodistal Oblique of the Navicular Bone (65°DP-conedown)

A. TECHNIQUE

The positioning for this view is similar for the 65°DP-P3, but the exposure factors are doubled, the beam is centered at the coronary band, and the collimation of the x-ray beam is greater (conedown). A general guideline regarding collimation of the beam is the exposure field should be a two by five inch area (proximal-distal by medial-lateral). The reason for collimation is to reduce scatter radiation resulting in increased radiographic detail. The properly positioned 65°DP-conedown will have the entire silhouette of the navicular bone superimposed on P2 with the distal border of the navicular bone proximal to both the joint space and the palmar border of proximal P3 (Figure 4-8).

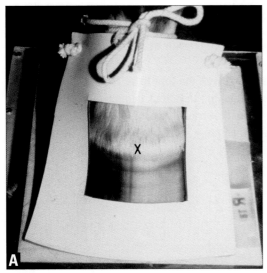
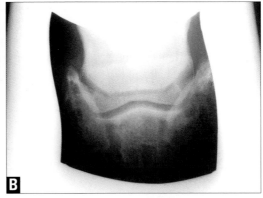

Figure 4-8. *The positioning for the 65°DP conedown is the same angulation as for the 65°DP-P3. The collimator is used to reduce the size of the field of exposure, i.e., conedown. A window cut into a small piece of an old lead apron can be used for collimation if an x-ray machine does not have a collimator (**A**). The resultant radiograph produced (**B**) demonstrates that this window could be reduced in size for the proximal to distal direction by about 30 percent. The exposure technique for this view is approximately twice that used for the 65°DP-P3.*

B. COMMON PROBLEMS

1. Poor cleaning and packing of the foot
2. The degree of angulation is not great enough to elevate the silhouette of the distal flexor border above the joint space and palmar margin of P3
3. Inadequate degree of collimation

C. ANATOMICAL AREAS EVALUATED

The 65°DP conedown is taken to evaluate the body and distal border of the navicular bone and the distal interphalangeal joint (Figure 4-9). It is not utilized to evaluate the proximal border of the navicular bone because productive change at the proximal border is distorted on this view. The 45°DP must be used to accurately evaluate change at the proximal border of the navicular bone. The width of the distal interphalangeal joint space plus the subchondral bone of distal P2 and proximal P3 are optimally seen on this DP projection. These anatomical areas can best be evaluated if the positioning permits the distal border of the navicular bone to be seen proximal to the palmar border of proximal P3.

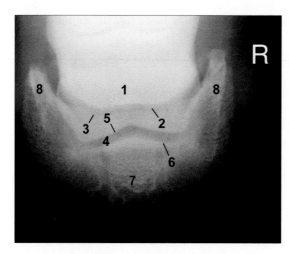

Figure 4-9. The 65°DP-conedown view permits optimum evaluation of the following anatomical areas:
- Distal one-half of the body of the navicular bone (1)
- Distal flexor border (2) of the navicular bone
- Palmar border of the third phalanx (3)
- Distal interphalangeal joint space (4) and the subchondral bone of the distal P2 (5) and proximal P3 (6)
- Proximal body (7) and heel regions (8) of P3

5. Extended Palmaro 50°Proximal-Palmarodistal Oblique (Flexor or Navicular Skyline View)

A. TECHNIQUE

This projection is produced using the cassette tunnel with the foot to be radiographed placed 12-14 inches behind that of the opposite limb resulting in the fetlock being hyper-extended (Figure 4-10). The view is taken with an x-ray beam that travels palmaroproximally to palmarodistally parallel to the slope of the pastern (approximately 50°) and centered at midline between the bulbs of the heels. Identification markers are placed adjacent to the lateral hoof wall within the collimated exposure field.

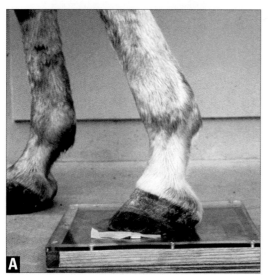
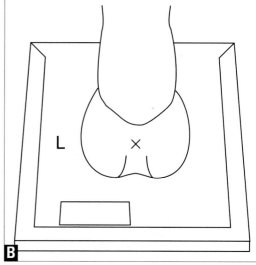

Figure 4-10. The skyline view of the navicular bone of the front limb is produced by an exposure made by an x-ray beam from the palmaro50°proximal to palmarodistal obliquity. The limb is extended in the palmar direction with the foot on a cassette tunnel *(A)*, and the beam is centered (X) on midline approximately two inches dorsally at the "shelf" formed by the heel region *(B)*.

B. COMMON PROBLEMS

1. Excluding this view as a part of the routine DEE
2. Foot is not placed far enough in extension
3. X-ray beam is not angled enough proximally
4. Poor foot preparation, especially inadequate cleaning and packing

C. ANATOMICAL AREAS EVALUATED

The navicular skyline view allows the flexor surface, flexor cortex, medullary cavity, and the navicular ridge of the navicular bone to be interpreted without superimposition of the second and third phalanges (Figure 4-11). The heel regions of P3, both the axial and abaxial surfaces, and the soft tissues of the palmar region of the foot are also best evaluated on this view. This view is an absolute requirement for the DEE of a horse with clinical signs compatible with caudal heel lameness.

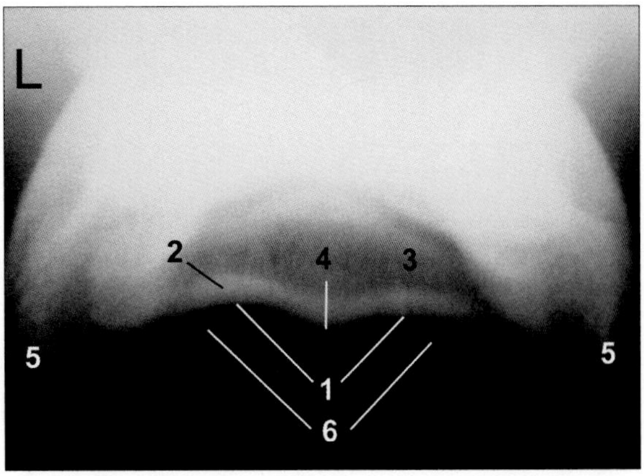

Figure 4-11. The skyline or flexor view permits optimum evaluation of the following anatomical areas:
• The flexor surface (1), cortex (2), and medullary cavity (3) of the navicular bone, and the navicular ridge (4)
• Heels of P3 (5)
• Palmar soft tissues (6)

3. Special Radiographic Projections of the Distal Extremity

It would seem that the five views of the routine DEE should be adequate to evaluate foot lameness. In most patients this is true, but in some a special projection can be very beneficial to interpretation. Two special projections can improve the diagnostic accuracy when evaluating the equine digit. These special views are the oblique heel (medial or lateral) and the horizontal DP projections.

1. Dorso 65°ProximoY°Lateral (Medial)-Palmarodistomedial (Lateral) Oblique (Oblique Heel Projections)

A. TECHNIQUE

The foot is placed on the cassette with identification markers to identify either the medial or lateral heel that is silhouetted. This view has compound angulation and can be described generically as a D65°PrY°M(L)-PaDiL(M)O. This generic description indicates both oblique views have the same degrees of angulation. It is important to realize the "rectangle" schematic of the structure of an anatomical area (see Chapter 5, IIB for a detailed explanation of this idea), because the medial and lateral heel views are taken to highlight palmar regions of the foot, but the descriptive terminology is named by the dorsal region highlighted. Therefore, the D65°PrY°M-PaDiLO is the "lateral oblique" but it highlights the palmaromedial aspect of the foot, while the D65°PrY°L-PaDiMO ("medial oblique") highlights the palmaro-lateral aspect of the foot. If the primary area to evaluate is the solar margin of P3, the abaxial obliquity is 60° and the exposure factors are similar to the 65°DP-P3. If an extremity change or avulsion fracture of the navicular bone is suspected, the abaxial obliquity is 45° and the exposure factors are similar to those for the 65°DP-conedown (Figure 4-12). Therefore, the first view highlighting the solar margin of P3 is described as a D65°Pr60°M(L)-PaDiL(M)O and the latter highlighting the abaxial region of the navicular bone is described as a D65°Pr45°M(L)-PaDiL(M)O.

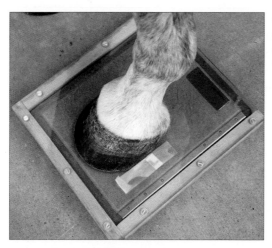

Figure 4-12. *A photograph demonstrates the positioning of the foot using the cassette tunnel to produce the oblique views of the solar margin of P3 and extremity of the navicular bone.*

B. COMMON PROBLEMS
1. Not taking the special view when a lesion is suspected from the routine DEE
2. Improper abaxial angulation and exposure for the anatomical region desired to be evaluated
3. Severe bilateral pain can result in the inability to produce this view!

C. ANATOMICAL AREAS EVALUATED (FIGURE 4-13)
The heel projections are taken primarily to evaluate either the extremity and distal abaxial regions of the navicular bone [(D65°Pr45°M(L)-PaDiL(M)O] or the solar border of the heel and quarter regions of P3 [D65°Pr60°M(L)-PaDiL(M)O].

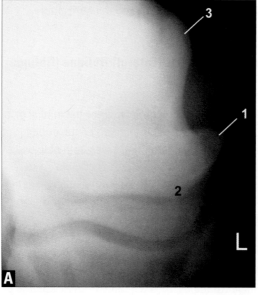
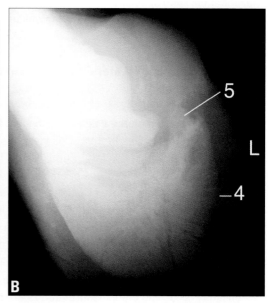

Figure 4-13. *The two oblique heel views are special views taken for optimum evaluation of the following anatomical areas:*
A. D65°Pr45°L(M)-PaDiM(L)O (A):
• Extremity (1) and distal abaxial (2) region of the navicular bone
• Palmaroproximal P2 (3)

B. D65°Pr60°M(L)-PaDiL(M)O (B):
• Solar margin of P3 in the heel and quarter regions (4)
• Palmar process of P3 in the heel region (5)

2. Dorso 0°Proximal-Palmarodistal Oblique (Extensor Process View)

A. TECHNIQUE

The foot is placed on the positioning block with the fetlock against a cassette and identification markers taped to the lateral aspect of the face of the cassette. The x-ray beam is centered on midline at the coronary band and directed perpendicular to the cassette resulting in a radiographic view described as a D0°Pr-PaDiO (Figure 4-14). The exposure factors are similar to the 65°DP-conedown view.

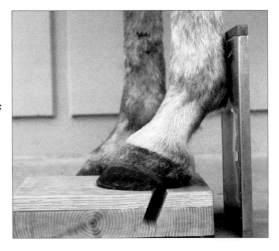

Figure 4-14. A photograph demonstrates the positioning of the foot to produce the extensor process view (D0°Pr-PaDiO). This view is a special view and should not be included as part of the routine DEE (i.e., instead of the 45°DP).

B. COMMON PROBLEMS

1. Including this view as part of a routine DEE instead of the 45°DP.
2. Not taking this special view when indicated by a suspected lesion seen with the routine DEE
3. Underexposure

C. ANATOMICAL AREAS EVALUATED

This projection is a special radiographic view for evaluating the equine distal extremity rather than a view in the routine DEE. Many AEP take this view instead of the 45°DP because it is easier to produce. However, the D0°Pr-PaDiO does not allow the proximal border or body of the navicular bone to be seen. This view allows the extensor process of P3, ossified collateral cartilages, the soft tissues distal to the solar margin for suspected subsolar gas (abscessation), and the relationship of P3 within the hoof capsule to be evaluated. The solar margin, DIP, and PIP should be parallel if the horse is properly trimmed and full weight-bearing when the radiograph was exposed (Figure 4-15).

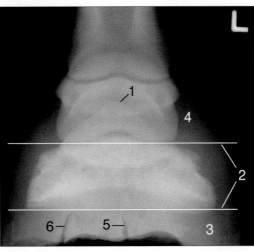

Figure 4-15. The extensor process or D0°Pr-PaDiO view is taken for optimum evaluation of the following anatomical areas:
• Extensor process of P3 (1) and the relationship of P3 within the hoof capsule (2) determined by the medial and lateral solar margins of P3 being parallel to the distal interphalangeal joint space.
• Soft tissues distal to the solar margin of P3 (3)
• Density change of the collateral cartilages (4)
• Note the gas in the central (5) and medial (6) sulci of the frog resulting from inadequate packing

V. Technique Settings for the Distal Extremity Examination

To provide background information on technique settings for each projection of the DEE, the following exposures are offered for the average size, mature horse. There will be variation with different clinical practices, but these times will provide a reference point. The imaging system for these exposure times is a 400 speed rare-earth system, and the exposures were made at 80 kVp at 15 mA. The film focal distances are 26 inches. The exception to this distance is for the flexor skyline view which is 20 inches. These techniques are for double screen systems. Double emulsion film is recommended for the AEP, but single emulsion film will provide better bone detail. The cost for this improvement in detail is greater exposure time and increased film cost. As a general statement, single emulsion film is more expensive (10-15%) than double emulsion film. The reason is the single emulsion film is considered a specialty item.

A. Average exposure time for each projection for a double emulsion film

65°DP-Conedown	0.16 sec.
65°DP-P3	0.08 sec.
45°DP	0.1 sec.
Lateromedial	0.1 sec.
Flexor	0.1 sec.

B. Average techniques for a single emulsion film

65°DP-Conedown	0.2 sec.
65°DP-P3	0.12 sec.
45°DP	0.14 sec.
Lateromedial	0.14 sec.
Flexor	0.14 sec.

The exposure factors for rigid and vinyl cassettes are comparable.

VI. Conclusions

Producing a high quality and complete DEE in the field can be done with regularity if the foot is properly prepared, the radiographic technique is correct, and the projections are positioned properly. By limiting technical errors the AEP will increase diagnostic accuracy leading to a better treatment plan and a more accurate prognosis. There will also be a financial benefit that can be significant (Chapter 2).

NOTES

NOTES

NOTES

NOTES

Chapter 5

Basic Information for Radiographic Interpretation of the Distal Extremity Examination

I. Introduction

II. Basic Parameters Required to Accurately Interpret the DEE
1. Placement of Radiographs on Viewboxes
2. Nomenclature
    A. General Information
    B. Obliquity Information
3. Identification of Basic Radiographic Findings

III. Bony Response
1. Productive
2. Destructive

IV. Application of Identified Radiographic Findings at Specific Anatomical Locations

V. Variables to Consider for Interpreting Abnormal Findings

I. Introduction

Veterinary education is deficient in radiology instruction for the AEP. Most curricula have a total of less than five lecture hours on equine radiology and the instruction commonly uses the "lookie-whoopee" technique for teaching radiographic interpretation. I believe that if one is to correctly interpret radiographs they must know what radiographic signs to look for and relate the findings to anatomical locations. This is the technique I will apply to the DEE leading to conclusions and impression about the diagnosis. The approach is very basic.

II. Basic Parameters Required to Accurately Interpret the DEE

1. Placement of Radiographs on Viewboxes

The radiographs must be placed on the viewboxes in a routine order and interpreted individually from left-to-right. This order is the LM, 45° DP, 65° DP-P3, 65° DP-conedown, and the flexor skyline views. In addition, the views must be placed so laterality is consistent, i.e., the medial and lateral aspect of all views except the LM must be in the same orientation. The radiographic quality of the DEE must next be determined. Any limitations for interpretation must be identified and corrected at this time. The limitations may be preparation, positioning, or production problems (discussed in Chapter 1).

2. Nomenclature
A. General Information

Interpretation requires a command of general terminology related to the anatomical area being evaluated. The extremities are described using the following:

- Cranial or dorsal
- Caudal or palmar/plantar
- Medial or lateral
- Proximal or distal
- Axial or abaxial
- Right or left
- Fore or hind

The term cranial changes to dorsal and caudal to palmar/plantar at the level of the antebrachio-carpal (radiocarpal) articulation in the forelimb and the tarsocrural (tibiotarsal) articulation in the hind limbs. The use of the terms "anterior" and "posterior" is to be avoided.

Combining descriptive terms is done in a specific order using the following rules:
- **Right or left precedes other terms.**
- **Cranial/dorsal and caudal/palmar (plantar) take precedence over medial or lateral.**
- **Proximal or distal take precedence over medial or lateral but not cranial/dorsal or caudal/palmar (plantar).**

This terminology order can be demonstrated using as an example a lesion located dorsally and medially on the right limb distal to the carpus. The location is described as right dorsomedial...not dorsomedial right or right mediodorsal.

B. Obliquity Information

Oblique radiographic projections complement the LM and DP views and can be described either by the dorsal profile that is silhouetted or the descriptive terminology method where the route the x-ray beam traveled is described from the position of the x-ray unit to cassette when the exposure was made. The dorsal silhouette method can be summarized schematically (Figure 5-1). An anatomical area being radiographed is represented figuratively by a rectangle with dorsal-palmar and medial-lateral aspects of the rectangle making the four parts. A "medial" oblique view highlights the dorsomedial aspect and the "lateral" oblique view highlights the dorsolateral aspect.

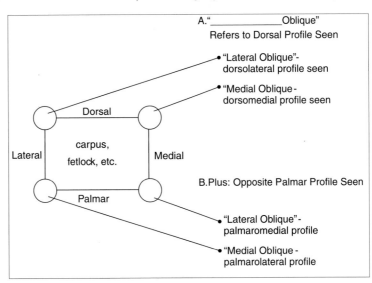

Figure 5-1. Summary of Oblique Projection Nomenclature. An oblique view is referred to by the dorsal profile that is highlighted (A). The opposite palmar profile is also highlighted (B).

It is important to emphasize that the opposite palmar (plantar) silhouette will be highlighted, e.g., the dorsomedial and palmarolateral for the "medial" oblique view. The specific axial to abaxial area highlighted depends on the degree of angulation from the dorsopalmar plane, i.e., the greater the angulation from DP up to ninety degrees, the closer the point silhouetted on the dorsomedial aspect will be towards midline (Figure 5-2).

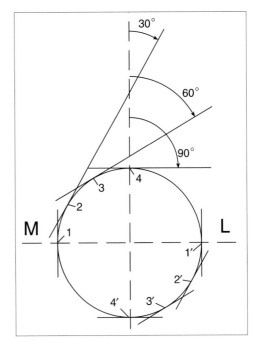

Figure 5-2. Abaxial angulation from the dorsopalmar plane results in different anatomical locations being highlighted radiographically on the dorsomedial region. This principle is demonstrated by lateral angulation of 0° (1), 30° (2), 60° (3), and 90°(4). The opposite palmar locations (lateral) are highlighted by these angulations, i.e., (1'), (2'), (3'), and (4'), respectively.

The specificity for angulation of oblique views is increased with the descriptive terminology method. This technique designates anatomically the relative positions of the x-ray unit and cassette at time of the exposure that produced a view. The rules related to this technique are:

- As the starting point, assume the x-ray unit is on the dorsopalmar plane and perpendicular to the examination site.
- The unit is first moved to the desired angulation (X°) in the proximal or distal direction.
- If there is no abaxial angulation, the view is described using these locations of the tube head and cassette. A generic example of this terminology for simple angulation is dorsox°proximal-palmarodistal oblique (DX°Pr-PaDiO).
- The descriptive terminology ends with the word "oblique" whenever the degrees of angulation are included. Only the LM view does not end in "oblique" for the DEE.
- If the exposure is made when the anatomical area is flexed or extended, the descriptive name is preceded by the word "flexed" or "extended."
- If there is abaxial angulation in addition to proximodistal angulation, the view is described as compound angulation. An example of compound angulation is dorso x°proximo y°medial-palmarodistolateral oblique (DX°PrY°M-PaDiLO) which is comparable to a lateral oblique using the other terminology, but the angulation provides precise information for replication.

The descriptive terminology will be used in the DEE and other anatomical areas to be more precise and develop reader familiarity to its use.

3. Identification of Basic Radiographic Findings

There are <u>six basic abnormal findings</u> that can be identified radiographically on the DEE. These findings may be identified individually or collectively, but it is the goal of the veterinarian to search for each finding on every radiographic view. **These findings are:**

A. Productive bony response
B. Destructive bony response
C Combination of productive-destructive response
D. Density change
   1) Decreased density (lucency)
     a. Linear
     b. Cystic
   2) Increased density
E. Contour irregularity
F. Increased soft tissue thickness

III. Bony Response

Bone responds to a stimulus producing radiographic findings that are productive, destructive, or a combination of productive and destructive. These findings are a result of increased osteoblastic and/or osteoclastic activity and can occur to varying degrees.

1. Productive Response

A productive bony finding in the horse is most commonly a result of stimulation to the periosteum (Figure 5-3). The stimulus can occur as a single incidence or more commonly as repeated events. A non-displaced fracture is an example of a single stimulus. Trauma to bone from interference (one limb striking another) is an example of repeated events producing a productive bony lesion. The actual injury probably results in tearing of the periosteum from the bone resulting in sub-periosteal hemorrhage and a stimulation of the osteoblasts in the periosteum. The severity of the stimulus, the anatomy of the periosteum, and the age of the patient are variables influencing the degree of periosteal response. These factors make establishment of the precise duration of a periosteal response almost impossible. This is particularly true for the third phalanx because the periosteum of P-3 becomes less complete and thins as it extends more distally. The periosteum of P-3 has been described as being complete proximally, but it becomes more like "screen wire" in the distal one-half of P-3 (R. R. Pool, Personal Communications). This lack of a well-defined periosteum distally explains the limited or lack of a periosteal productive response associated with solar margin fractures and infections.

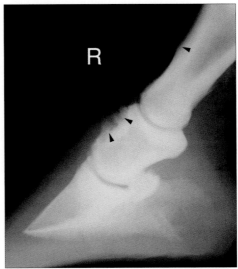

Figure 5-3. A productive periosteal response (arrowheads) is present on the dorsum of P2 (severe) and P1 (mild). This common radiographic finding usually indicates that the bone is responding to a traumatic injury. There are also productive periarticular changes at the dorsum of the proximal (PIP) and distal (DIP) interphalangeal joints.

A productive bony response seen at the site of a ligamentous or tendinous attachment is called an enthesophyte and it is a form of traumatic periosteitis (Figure 5-4). This productive bony response is commonly seen on the DEE at the palmar region of the mid-diaphysis of P-1 (insertion of the middle ligaments of the distal ligaments of the proximal sesamoid bones), the extensor process of P-3 (insertion of the common digital extensor tendon), and the proximal border of the navicular bone (insertion of the proximal suspensory ligaments of the navicular bone).

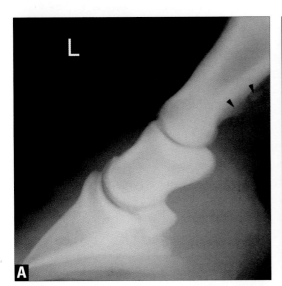 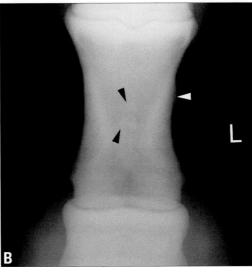

Figure 5-4. An enthesophyte with soft tissue calcification (arrowheads) of the middle of the distal ligaments of the proximal sesamoid bones is seen on the palmar aspect of P1 **(A)** near midline **(B)**. A smooth productive periosteal response is identified on the lateral surface of mid P1 (white arrowhead).

Productive bony responses are also identified on the DEE at the joint margins (Figure 5-5). These periarticular productive changes are referred to as periarticular osteophytes or remodeling changes. These findings are a result of a productive response where the joint cartilage thins and where the fibrous and synovial lining parts of the joint capsule attach to the bone. It is neither important, nor is it possible in most cases, whether the productive changes are originating from the joint capsule attachments or the articular margin. The important determination is how far the productive remodeling changes extend onto the joint surface. This determination is identified by irregularity to the subchondral surface and underlying sclerosis. It is also important to understand that the stimuli for periarticular productive change commonly cannot be determined radiographically, especially as the degree of these findings becomes greater and more extensive in location. This is why the term "secondary joint disease" (SJD) is recommended as the clinical diagnosis. SJD is a broad term that includes degenerative, infectious, and developmental etiologies responsible for the radiographic findings seen.

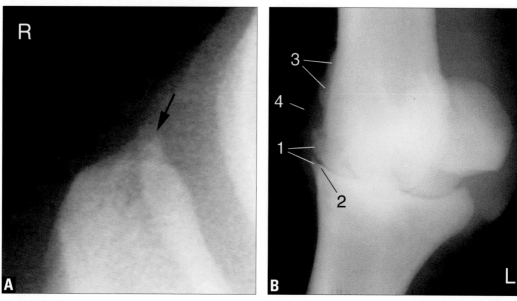

Figure 5-5. *Productive bony response at the joint margin (arrow) is referred to as a periarticular osteophyte and is compatible with secondary joint disease (A). This marginal remodeling change of the joint in the more chronic stages (B) commonly is accompanied by periarticular remodeling across the joint (1) with subchondral sclerosis (2), periosteal reaction (3), and joint capsule distention (4).*

2. Destructive Response

A loss of bone or osteolysis can result from excessive osteoclastic activity. This can be seen in the horse DEE as either a generalized effect or as a focal area of involvement. The generalized effect is seen commonly with disuse in the high performance horse with a fracture resulting in a non-weight bearing lameness (Figure 5-6). In seven to ten days there will be generalized demineralization seen on the DEE involving the phalanges and especially the proximal sesamoid bones. The trabecular pattern becomes more coarse in these bones secondary to a generalized osteoclastic response.

Osteolysis is also identified radiographically as decreased density especially when the osteoclastic activity is focal. The focal destructive change results from hyperemia which creates activation of osteoclasts. This effect is best seen radiographically at the periarticular region of

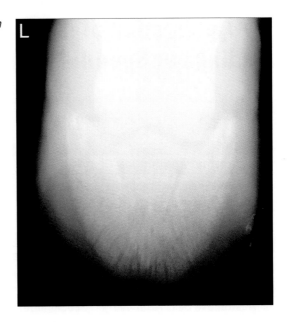

Figure 5-6. A generalized destruction of bone is often seen in the distal extremity of the high performance horse that suffers a fracture. The trabecular pattern becomes more coarse within 7-10 days secondary to the osteoclastic response.

palmarodistal MCIII (Figure 5-7). The net effect of this hyperemic effect is a remodeling of the MCIII in this area producing a condition called supracondylar lysis. This destructive change is also associated with a change in contour in the remodeled area.

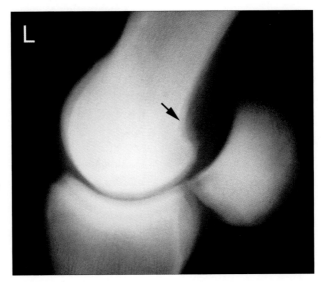

Figure 5-7. A focal destructive lesion results from a local hyperemia which stimulates osteoclastic activity. Supracondylar lysis at the palmarodistal MCIII results from this change and is identified radiographically by signs of the focal cortical destruction and alteration of the contour (arrow).

A focal destructive lesion of the third phalanx often results from infection. The lesion results from osteolysis produced by osteoclastic activity and the acidic effect of the exudate. This type of lesion involving the solar margin can be identified radiographically as a result of a destructive bony response, a focal area of decreased density, and a contour irregularity. This lesion and supracondylar lysis demonstrates how identification of combinations of these six basic radiographic findings are important in establishing the radiographic diagnosis.

IV. Application of Identified Basic Radiographic Findings at Specific Anatomical Locations

The identification of these six findings (see II-3) at <u>specific anatomical locations</u> can be related to clinical diagnoses as indicated below:

Abnormal Finding	Location	Clinical Diagnoses
A. Productive bony response	Periosteal	Traumatic periosteitis or periosteitis secondary to infection
	Periarticular	Secondary joint disease
	Site of ligament or tendinous attachment	Enthesophytosis (traumatic periosteitis)
B. Destructive bony response	Subchondral	OCD, osteoarthrosis, osteomyelitis, or infectious arthritis
	Cortex	Osteomyelitis, Chronic fracture, neoplasia (rare), and osteonecrosis
	Medullary	Chronic osteomyelitis, fracture, or OCD
	Combination of above locations	Osteomyelitis, chronic fracture, or OCD
C. Combination productive/ destructive bony responses	Periosteal, cortical, or medullary	Osteomyelitis, chronic fracture, neoplasia (rare)

D. Density change
  1. Decreased density (lucency)
  • Cystic (Figure 5-8)
	Subchondral	OCD, chronic incomplete fracture, osteoarthrosis, subchondral cyst, or packing artifact

	Within the navicular bone	Navicular degeneration, fracture site, osteomyelitis, or packing artifact
	Within the third phalanx	Osteomyelitis, packing artifact, keratoma (rare), or vascular abnormality (rarer)
• Linear (Figure 5-9)	Within a single bone	Fracture (complete or incomplete), nutrient canal, or packing artifact
	Within multiple bones	Packing artifact
	Within soft tissues	Cellulitis, laminitis, packing artifact

2. Increased density	On skin surface	Debris
	Within soft tissues	Fracture fragment, soft tissue calcification, dense foreign body, or artifact
E. Contour irregularity (asymmetry)	Subchondral	Fracture, OCD, osteomyelitis/infectious arthritis
	Solar margin	Fracture, infection, inflammation
	Cortex	Fracture, infection
F. Increased soft tissue thickness	Dorsal to P3 (>18mm)	Laminitis: with or without rotation, cold-blooded breeds
	Proximal to the coronary band	Cellulitis, trauma, or circulatory impairment

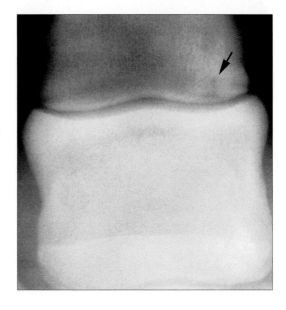

Figure 5-8. Cystic lucent changes associated with decreased density (arrow) are commonly identified in the subchondral and navicular bone.

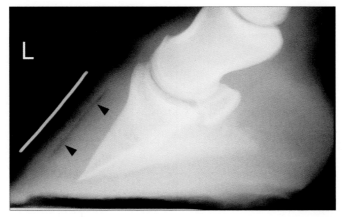

Figure 5-9. Linear lucent change may be seen within a single bone, multiple bones, or soft tissues. The most common clinical problem associated with a linear lucency in a single bone is a fracture, and within the soft tissue it is gas seen secondary to laminitis (arrowheads).

The radiographic technique used to precisely locate a radiographic finding in an anatomical area is called the "Law of the Circle." A finding is identified on the LM and DP (Figure 5-10A, B) radiographs (orthogonal views) and related to a circle which figuratively represents a cross-section of the area with the findings (Figure 5-10C). On any one view the finding identified could be located from one skin surface to the opposite skin surface. The orthogonal view is interpreted and the finding can also be located from one skin surface to the opposite. The point where the two lines intersect within the circle is where the finding is actually located in the patient. Oblique views are used to evaluate the area for additional radiographic signs (Figure 5-10D, E).

In summary, the identification of the basic abnormal findings individually or collectively is the diagnostic key to interpreting radiographic examinations associated with foot lameness resulting from disorders of the hoof wall, phalanges, navicular bone, and interphalangal joints.

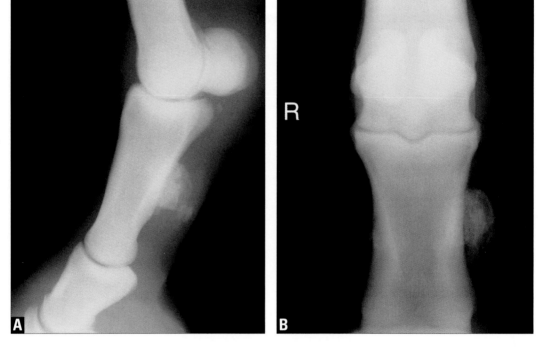

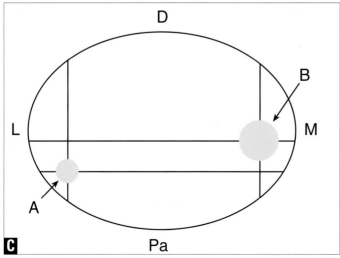

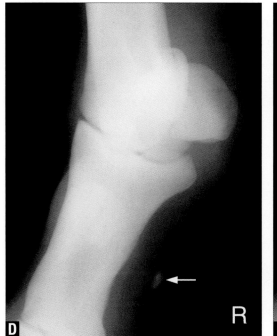
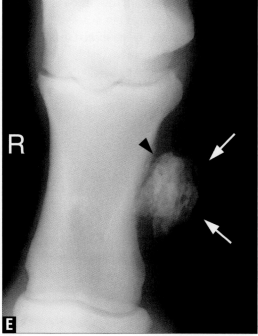

Figure 5-10. *Increased density within soft tissues may represent soft tissue calcification. The orthogonal views (LM and DP) must be interpreted first to establish that the densities are within the soft tissues (**A, B**). The radiographic interpretation must include the precise localization of the density and this is done using the "Law of the Circle" (**C**). The smaller density is palmarolaterally and the larger density is palmaromedially. The oblique views confirm there are two calcific densities as seen on the DP and they are not on the skin surface (**D, E**). Note the larger density has produced a contour change at the surface and extends deeply producing a periosteal response at the palmaromedial surface of the right P1 (arrowhead).*

V. Variables to Consider for Interpreting Abnormal Findings

It is important to emphasize that the **entire** DEE must be interpreted. Change(s) or suspected change(s) seen on one projection must be evaluated on all views of the DEE for complete assessment leading to an accurate radiographic conclusion (Figure 5-11). The radiographic findings must be correlated to the clinical history and examination. However, it is strongly advised that the radiographs be interpreted before this correlation is done. This will avoid errors of omission which are common in interpreting equine radiographs.

The degree of the findings may vary from focal to extensive, active to inactive, mild to severe, and non-significant to highly significant. Radiographic interpretation first involves identification of abnormal findings followed by careful analysis of these variables. **It is important to emphasize that some radiographic findings may not be associated with clinical signs. This occurs most commonly when the findings are focal, inactive, and of a mild degree.**

In summary, this chapter provides basic information for interpreting radiographic examinations of the distal extremity and other anatomical areas. **The six basic radiographic findings in specific anatomical locations is the format for the AEP to follow for interpreting all radiographic examinations in the horse.**

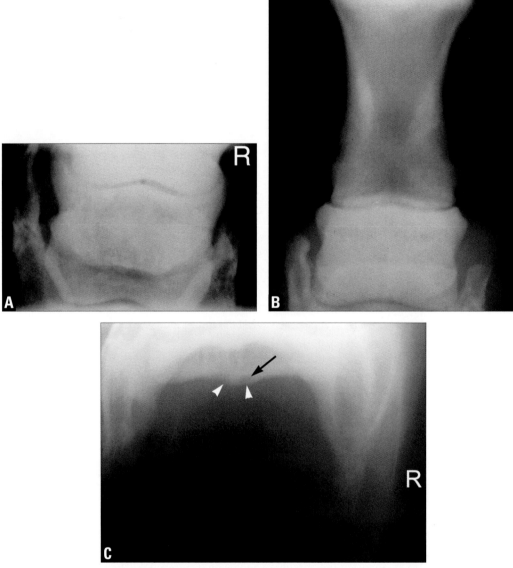

Figure 5-11. *The importance of careful interpretation and correlation of radiographic findings on all views can be demonstrated using the DEE of an 8-year old Quarter Horse with clinical signs compatible with bilateral navicular disease that were more evident on the right front. Cystic lucencies can be identified in the right navicular bone on the 65°DP conedown (**A**), but the lucencies were not as evident in the mid-body of the navicular bone on the 45°DP (**B**). The LM (see Figure 5-3) was interpreted and there were extensive periosteal productive changes on the dorsum of P2 as well as periarticular productive change at the dorsum of the PIP and DIP joints. The concern was whether the cystic lucencies in the navicular bone identified on the 65°DP conedown resulted from superimposition of the dorsal P2 changes, i.e., was there really degeneration of the navicular bone? Interpretation of the skyline flexor view (**C**) documented surface contour irregularity (white arrowheads) and flexor cortical lucency (black arrow) compatible with degeneration of the navicular bone. There is also extensive ossification of the collateral cartilages with the degree being greater in the medial than the lateral collateral cartilage (**A, B**).*

NOTES

NOTES

NOTES

NOTES

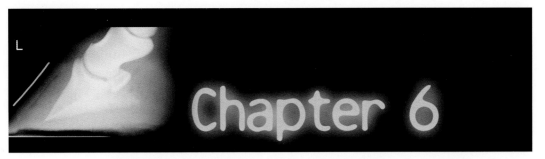

Radiographic Interpretation of the Third Phalanx, Hoof Wall, and Soft Tissue Structures in the Foot

I. Introduction

The third phalanx is evaluated radiographically primarily with the LM and 65° DP-P3. The other three views of the routine DEE contribute some information but diagnostic evaluation of P3 using these three views is limited to localized areas. Interpretation of P3 for abnormalities is based on identification of the six basic abnormal findings (signs) discussed in the Chapter 5. This chapter deals with the identification of these six changes in specific anatomical locations associated with the third phalanx and hoof wall as they appear on the radiographic views of the DEE.

II. Lateromedial View in Evaluating the Third Phalanx and Soft Tissues of the Distal Extremity

1. Extensor Process (EP)

The dorsoproximal P3 has a bony prominence (EP) with a smooth dorsal surface. The common digital (front) and long digital (hind) extensor tendons insert on this protuberance. Closely associated with the palmar (plantar) aspect of the EP are the dorsal periarticular region of the DIP joint and the subchondral bony surface of P3 (Figure 6-1). A correlation of the radiographic findings in these anatomical areas to the clinical diagnosis can be made from the LM view.

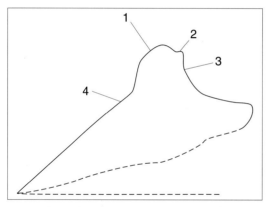

Figure 6-1. The extensor process (EP) appears as a smooth bony prominence at the dorsoproximal P3 (1). The periarticular (2) and subchondral surface of P3 (3) are seen palmar to the EP, and distal to the EP is the straight dorsal cortex of P3 (4).

Area	Change	Radiographic Conclusion(s)
A. Extensor Process	**Periosteal productive**	**Enthesophytosis**
	Linear lucency	**Fracture**
	Density: Increased (proximal to the EP)*	**Displaced facture** **Dystrophic calcification**
B. Dorsal Periarticular	**Productive (see Figure 5-5A)**	**Secondary joint disease**
	Combination productive-destructive	**Secondary joint disease**
C. Subchondral Bone of P3	**Cystic lucency***	**Bone cyst** **OCD** **Chronic incomplete fracture**
	Linear lucency*	**Fracture**

*Action: A D0°Pr-PaDiO is indicated for more complete evaluation of this change.

2. Dorsal Cortex of P3 and Hoof Wall

The dorsal cortex of the front P3 should have a straight, smooth surface extending from an indentation just distal to the EP to the toe of P3. The hind P3 often has a slight dorsal convexity with a smooth surface. The cortex varies from a thin, straight dense line in the horse performing at a low level of athletic activity to a thick dense cortex in the horse performing at a high level of athletic activity (e.g., racehorse). The thickest region is located in the middle one-third of the dorsal cortex and the inner aspect appears bowed (thickened) palmarly (Figure 6-2). The distal one-fourth of the dorsal cortex can appear as a uniform thickness and density or have a linear lucency extending from the toe proximally for a few centimeters. This linear lucency is a normal dishing variant created by the crena in the toe of the P3. The dorsal hoof wall thickness is measured from the surface of the dorsal cortex to the surface of the hoof wall. A radiodense wire should be taped on the dorsal hoof wall prior to the exposure to assist in this measurement. This wire (about 2-3 inches) should extend from the toe to the junction of the proximal and middle one-third of the dorsal hoof wall. The wire should not extend to the coronary band because this will create errors in measuring if the hoof is dished proximally.

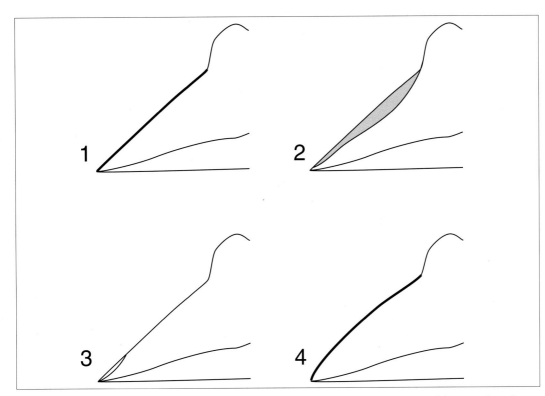

Figure 6-2. The radiographic appearance of the dorsal cortex of the normal P3 has a straight, smooth surface and varies in thickness related to the level of athletic performance from a thin (1) to a thick cortex (2). The former is expected in the low performance horse and the latter is seen in high performance horses. The distal one-fourth of the dorsal cortex can have a linear lucency (3) created by the crena. The dorsal cortex of P3 in the hind limbs tends to have a slight dorsal convexity but the dorsal surface is smooth (4).

Measurements should be made at two points, i.e., one proximally and one distally, to determine the dorsal hoof wall thickness. The two points for measurement are recommended to be at 25% and 75% of the total length of the straight-part of the dorsal cortex of P3 which is from toe to just distal to the EP (Figure 6-3). These two points are not absolute, e.g., they could be at 30% and 80% of the total length, but the points must be at consistent locations to establish if there is a difference. It is important that the distal measurement not be made from the toe so artifacts

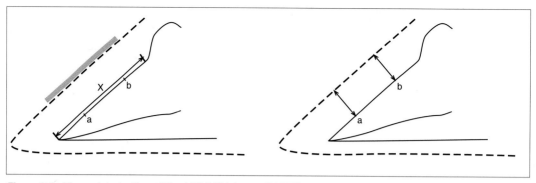

Figure 6-3. *Measuring the Dorsal Hoof Wall Thickness (DHWT):*
1. "X" is the total length of the straight part of the dorsal cortex of P3.
2. Point "a" is at 25% of "X".
3. Point "b" is at 75% of "X".
A wire is taped on the surface of the dorsal hoof wall to permit an accurate measurement to be made from the LM radiograph.

created in horses with a long toe will be avoided. The interpretation of the measurement data is based on either a difference between the proximal and distal (laminitis with rotation) or an increased thickness (greater than 18 mm) for breeds excluding cold-blooded breeds (Figure 6-4). Normal hoof wall thickness is 18 mm or less (commonly it is 16 mm) and the two measurements are equal. An increased thickness is a result of swelling of the laminae, and when the thickness measurements are different and the distal is greater, breakdown of the laminae and rotation are indicated. Two recommendations are suggested to increase the value of this radiographic determination: 1) Radiograph both feet for comparison measurements; and 2) Carefully evaluate the dorsal cortex of P3 for signs of productive bony change (associated with tearing of the insertions of the laminae into P3) seen with chronicity.

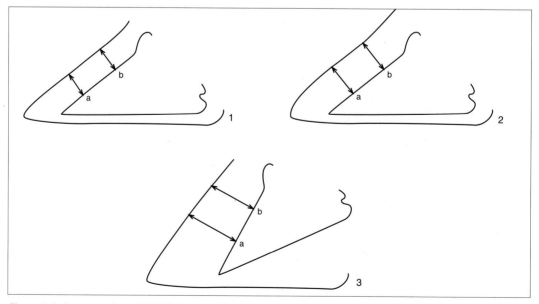

Figure 6-4. *Interpretation of DHWT for Laminitis.*
1. No evidence of Laminitis (1): DHWT at "a" and "b" are equal and less than 18 mm (16 mm for most common breeds of horses).
2. Laminitis without Rotation (2): DHWT at "a" and "b" are equal but greater than 18 mm.
3. Laminitis with Rotation (3): DHWT at "a" is greater than "b" and greater than 18 mm.

This productive change involving the middle and proximal one-thirds of dorsal P3 is compatible with a systemic cause of laminitis while this change limited to the distal one-third accompanied by a long toe is more compatible with a local mechanical cause (i.e. "road founder").

Correlations of radiographic findings in the dorsal hoof wall and dorsal cortex of P3 to the clinical diagnosis can be made from the LM radiographic evaluation.

Area	Change	Radiographic Conclusion(s)
A. Dorsal Hoof Wall	Increased thickness (>18mm), proximally and distally equal	Laminitis without rotation
	Increased thickness (>18mm), greater distally than proximally	Laminitis with rotation
	Linear lucency (gas) parallel to dorsal hoof wall (Figure 6-5)	Infection from a sole abscess Gas from a vacuum effect or a "poor man's arthrogram" effect
	Focal increased density dorsal or dorsoproximal to toe at solar margin (Figure 6-6)	Solar margin fracture Artifact associated with nail track
B. Dorsal Cortex of P3	Productive (Figure 6-7)	Chronic laminitis with or without rotation
	Destructive or destructive/ productive	Laminitis with osteomyelitis Osteomyelitis Keratoma (rare)
	Linear lucency in toe	Fracture Gas artifact Crena (normal)
	Contour at the toe (loss of sharp angle formed at the junction of dorsal and solar cortices Figure 6-8)	Chronic laminitis Chronic fracture Osteomyelitis

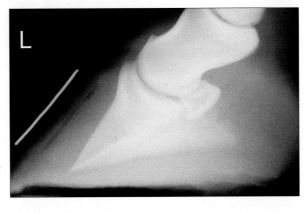

Figure 6-5. *A linear lucency parallel to the dorsal hoof wall seen on the LM radiograph is created by gas accumulating palmar to the insensitive lamina in this horse having laminitis with rotation of P3. A careful clinical examination of the sole in the toe region should be done for evidence of infection.*

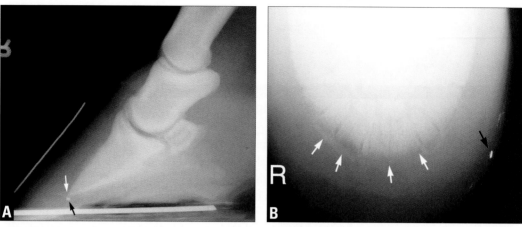

Figure 6-6. *A focal increased density dorsal or dorsoproximal to the toe of P3 seen on the LM radiograph (**A**) is commonly seen with laminitis. The density results from a solar margin fracture (white arrow) and/or an artifact associated with a nail track (black arrow). The degree of density and location seen on the 65°DP-P3 (**B**) demonstrates the very dense object is a medial hoof wall artifact. Extensive solar margin fractures (arrows) are seen dorsally and extending medially and laterally as a complication of laminitis with rotation.*

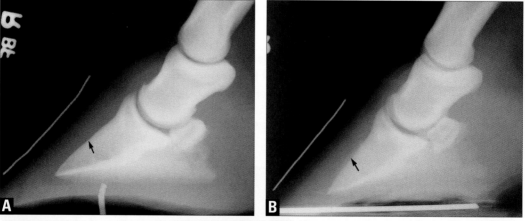

Figure 6-7. *Thickening of the dorsal hoof wall (19 mm at points "a" and "b") without rotation was determined for a horse with acute signs of foot lameness (**A**). The slightly undulating dorsal surface to P3 (arrow) is compatible with prior laminitis in this foot. At six months there is evidence of rotation and productive change (arrow) on the dorsal cortex of P3 (**B**).*

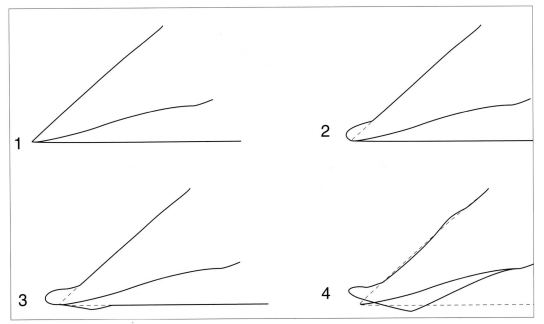

Figure 6-8. Remodeling changes (2-4) at the toe region of the normal P3 (1) secondary to chronic laminitis, fractures, and infection can be identified as an alteration of the contour of the toe region of P3 resulting in a "ski tip" appearance.).

3. Solar Margin of P3 and Solar Horny Tissues

The solar margin of P3 in the mature horse should appear as a smooth, arcuate bony surface extending from the toe to heel regions. Change in shape of the solar margin is best evaluated radiographically with other views of the DEE but this finding can be seen with chronic foot problems particularly remodeling secondary to laminitis, large toe fractures, infection, a club foot, and poor hoof care.

The solar horny tissues should appear as a homogenous soft tissue density that is slightly dished proximally. Gas shadows should be absent following packing, but in deeply dished feet, the use of more packing material may result in increased density in the frog region.

Area	Change	Radiographic Conclusion(s)
A. Solar Margin of P3	Contour: Flattening of solar area of toe secondary to remodeling	Chronic laminitis Chronic, large fractures Chronic infection Club foot conformation
	Combination destructive/productive	Osteomyelitis from a penetrating wound
B. Solar Horny Tissues	Lucency*	Sub-solar gas (abscess) Artifact: packing

*Action: A D0°Pr-PaDiO and the D65°Pr60°M(L)-PaDiL(M)O (oblique heel view) that highlights the region of the subsolar lucency are indicated for more complete evaluation of this finding.

4. Other Anatomical Areas

The angle of the heels, collateral cartilages, and the soft tissues in the heel region palmar (plantar) to the navicular bone are other areas that can be seen on the LM. However, these areas are better evaluated on other views of the DEE. In practice, these areas are interpreted from the views that permit better assessment and then the findings are located and evaluated on all views for the most complete interpretation.

III. Dorso65°Proximal-PalmaroDistal Oblique for P3 (65°DP-P3) in Evaluating the Third Phalanx and Soft Tissues of the Distal Extremity

The 65°DP-P3 view is the primary view to evaluate the solar border, vascular foramina, and trabecular detail of P3. It has very limited value in assessing the other phalanges, the interphalangeal joints, or the navicular bone. Overexposure of the 65° DP-P3 is a major problem for the AEP. Overexposure commonly results in an inability to visualize the solar margin of P3 and associated horny tissues. The average AEP should reduce exposure time for the 65° DP-P3 by a factor of at least two and probably four (Figure 6-9).

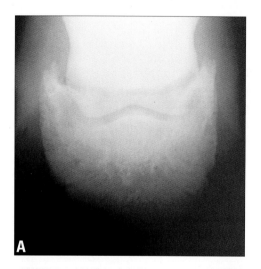
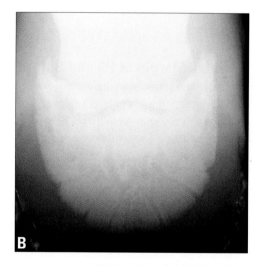
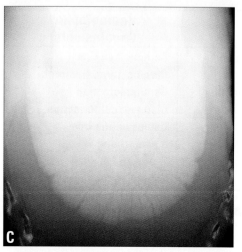

Figure 6-9. A major radiographic problem for the AEP is the solar margin of P3 cannot be interpreted because of over-exposure (*A*). A reduction in exposure time by a factor of two (*B*) or four (*C*) will correct this technical problem.

1. Solar Border and Body of P3

The solar margin of P3 is subdivided into the heel, quarter, and toe regions. Interpretation of the solar margin can be assisted by placing a curvilinear line with a grease pencil on the radiograph at the solar margin extending from the heel to toe. The ideal solar margin should have a contour that is similar to this line and the vascular foramina should touch this line. The bone at a foramen should form a 90° angle between that of the wall of the vascular canal and the solar border (Figure 6-10). Remodeling change at the solar margin is identified by bony resorption at the foramina resulting in widening and a serrated appearance to the solar margin. In the active stages of this remodeling process, the trabecular pattern will become more coarse. The entire solar margin must be evaluated for these remodeling changes because the changes in the more active stages are often confined to a focal area or region. Detailed clinical examination with hoof tester should follow to correlate evidence of a painful response to the location of radiographic findings. This clinical correlation is extremely valuable because the ability of P3 to remodel is limited at the solar margin (associated with the lack of a complete periosteum). Once the solar border becomes irregular there is an inability to regain the smooth contour. However, the trabecular structure will return to a finer detail.

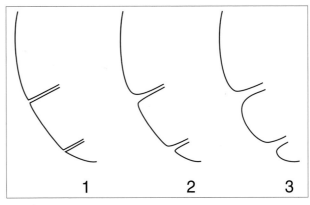

Figure 6-10. *The contour of the normal solar margin should appear smooth with vascular foramina at the solar margin forming a 90° angle (1). Remodeling change at the solar margin involving the vascular foramen produces an irregular solar margin contour. Resorption of bone at the vascular foramen results in widening of the foramen and the vascular canal (2 and 3).*

Area	Change	Radiographic Conclusion(s)
A. Solar Margin of P3*	**Radiodense body or bodies**	**Fracture(s)** **Artifact(s): cleaning**
	Irregular contour **(Figure 6-11)**	**Inflammation (pedal osteitis)** **Resorption of Fractures**
	Density loss of trabecular bone	**Osteopenia due to inflammation or disuse**
	Combination destructive/ productive	**Osteomyelitis** **Chronic fracture**
B. Body of P3*	**Linear lucency**	**Fracture** **Artifact: packing**
	Cystic lucency	**Chronic osteomyelitis** **Keratoma** **Artifact: packing**
	Multiple, very small lucencies	**End-on vascular canals in the dorsal cortex secondary to laminitis with rotation**
	Combination destructive/ productive	**Osteomyelitis** **Keratoma**

*Action: D65°Pr60°M(L)-PaDiL(M)O views that highlight the solar margin and body of P3 in the region of change on the routine DEE are indicated for more complete evaluation of changes in these areas before reaching a conclusion.

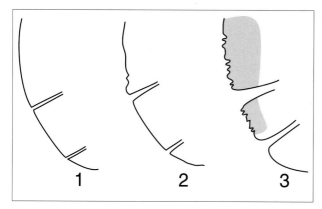

Figure 6-11. The contour of the normal, smooth solar margin of P3 (1) can become irregular secondary to inflammation (2) or resorption of a solar margin fracture. The adjacent trabecular bony pattern of P3 will appear more coarse (shading) indicating resorption and a loss of bone density (3).

2. Hoof Wall and Sole

The 65° DP-P3 must have a reduced exposure to visualize the hoof wall and sole. Hoof wall defects and gas accumulation can be evaluated with this view.

IV. Dorso65°Proximal-PalmaroDistal Oblique Conedown (65°DP Conedown) in Evaluating the Third Phalanx and Soft Tissues of the Distal Extremity

The 65° DP conedown view is primarily utilized to evaluate the navicular bone. It is used to complement the 65° DP-P3 for evaluating the third phalanx because it allows the subchondral bone and the bony trabecular pattern in proximal P3 to be seen in greater detail (Figure 6-12).

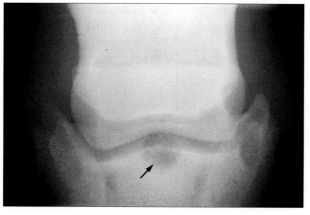

Figure 6-12. The 65°DP conedown allows the subchondral bone and trabecular pattern of proximal P3 to be evaluated. A subchondral cystic lucency in P3 (arrow) was identified in a horse with a chronic low-grade foot lameness.

Area	Change	Radiographic Conclusion(s)
A. Subchondral bone and trabecular pattern of proximal P3	Linear lucency*	Fracture Artifact: packing
	Cystic lucency*	Articular fracture Subchondral cyst Artifact: packing

*Action: A D0°Pr-PaDiO view is indicated for more complete evaluation of change in this area before reaching a conclusion.

V. Dorso45°Proximal-PalmaroDistal Oblique (45°DP) in Evaluating the Third Phalanx and Soft Tissues of the Distal Extremity

There is limited diagnostic value to evaluating the third phalanx with the 45° DP. The distal interphalangeal joint (DIJ) space width, ossified collateral cartilages, and the vertical foot axis can be interpreted, but the third phalanx is better evaluated on the dorsopalmar plane with the 65° DP-P3 and the 65° DP-Conedown.

VI. Extended Palmaro50°Proximal-PalmaroDistal Oblique (Flexor Skyline) in Evaluating the Third Phalanx and Soft Tissues of the Distal Extremity

The third phalanx evaluation using the flexor skyline view is limited to the heel regions. The heels are evaluated for linear lucencies associated with a fracture and productive change on the axial and abaxial surfaces of the heels. The soft tissues in the heel region can also be evaluated. This evaluation is important in determining if an increased density seen on the LM view is within the soft tissue of the heel region (calcification) or on the hoof wall surface (cleaning artifact).

VII. The Role of Special Radiographic Views in Evaluating the Third Phalanx and Soft Tissues of the Distal Extremity

1. Dorso0°Proximal-PalmaroDistal Oblique View
The D0°Pr-PaDiO view is supplemental to evaluating the P3 and soft tissues of the foot. This view is taken to obtain additional diagnostic information regarding the extensor process, solar margin of P3, ossified collateral cartilages, and solar soft tissues (Figure 6-13). The radiographic changes and associated radiographic conclusions associated with these areas are summarized.

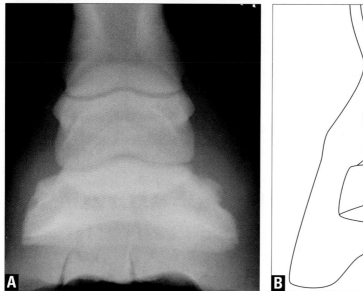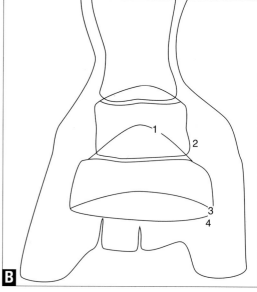

Figure 6-13. *The dorso0°proximal-palmarodistal oblique view is supplemental to the DEE **(A)**. Additional information can be determined regarding contour and density findings **(B)** at the extensor process (1), the area of the collateral cartilages (2), solar margins of P3 (3), and the solar soft tissues (4). Note there is gas in the medial and central sulci of the frog secondary to inadequate packing.*

Area	Change	Radiographic Conclusion(s)
A. Extensor process	Contour defect	Avulsion fracture Secondary joint disease
B. Solar margin of P3	Density: lucency	Infection Fracture with resorption
	Medial and lateral differential in position of solar margins	Breakdown within the hoof capsule
C. Collateral cartilages	Density: increased	Ossification of collateral cartilages
	Density: lucent region in ossified cartilages	Dystrophic calicification and incomplete ossification
	Narrow horizontal lucent region in ossified cartilages with bony production bridging the lucency	Fracture with healing
D. Solar soft tissues	Density: lucency (gas) adjacent to palmar aspect of the solar margin and body of P3	Subsolar infection (abscess)
	Thickness variation between medial and lateral	Broken M-L foot axis

2. Dorso65°Proximo60°Medial (Lateral)-PalmaroDistoLateral (Medial) Oblique

The oblique heel views of P3 allow the solar margin, palmar process, and trabecular pattern in the heel and quarter regions to be evaluated in greater detail (Figure 6-14). The 65°DP-P3 view is complemented by the oblique heel views where there are suspected changes in P3 and artifacts. Comparing these two views commonly permits confirmation of the presence or absence of a suspected radiographic change by their relative positions. The radiographic changes and associated radiographic conclusions for the P3 areas highlighted are summarized.

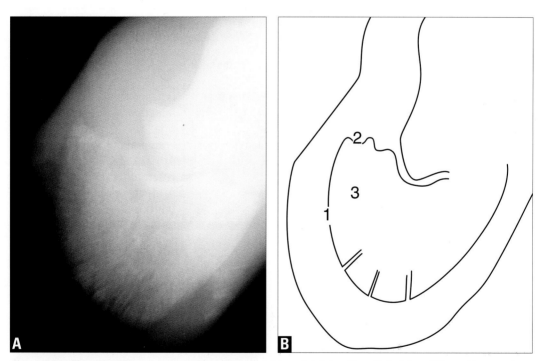

Figure 6-14. *The dorso65°proximo60°medial (lateral)-palmarodistolateral (medial) oblique **(A)** provides supplemental diagnostic information to findings suspected on the 65° DP conedown and P3 views at the solar margin (1), palmar process (2), and about the trabecular pattern (3) in the heel and quarter regions **(B)**.*

Area	Change	Radiographic Conclusion(s)
A. Solar margin	Density: lucency	Infection Fracture site following resorption Artifact: packing
	Density: dense body	Fracture Artifact: cleaning or post packing
	Contour: irregular	Inflammation (pedal osteitis) Fracture Infection
	Destructive	Infection Artifact: packing
B. Trabecular pattern	Destruction	Infection Artifact: packing Fracture with infection Keratoma
	Combination destruction-production	Infection Chronic fracture with infection
	Density: generalized reduction (coarser trabecular pattern)	Disuse osteopenia
	Density: focal reduction	Inflammation Infection
C. Palmar process	Density: linear lucency	Fracture Artifact: packing
	Destructive	Fracture Artifact: packing Infection

VIII. Fractures of the Third Phalanx

1. Introduction

The radiographic signs associated with P3 fractures in specific anatomical locations as seen on different views of the DEE has been described in the veterinary literature. In summary, third phalanx fractures can be identified as linear lucencies, separate dense bodies, associated with an irregular contour, or by a combination destructive-productive change. These radiographic signs tend to be associated with specific anatomical areas (Figure 6-15).

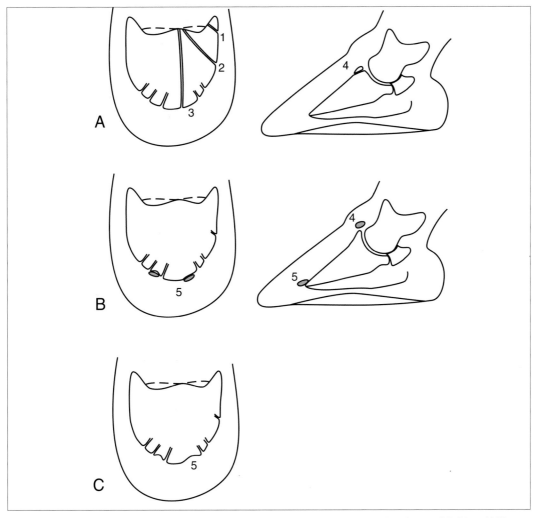

Figure 6-15. *Third phalanx fractures are commonly identified radiographically using the 65° DP-P3 and LM radiographs as linear lucencies (A), separate dense bodies (B), or associated with irregular solar contour (C). These radiographic findings tend to be associated with specific anatomical locations, and are described as Types I (1), II (2), III (3), IV (4), V and VI (5) fractures. The palmar process fracture described in Figure 6-17 has been classified as a Type VII.*

Radiographic Sign	Anatomical Area
A. Linear lucency (lucencies)	Body of P3 Heel of P3 Body of EP
B. Dense body (bodies)	Solar margin Proximal to EP Dorsoproximal to the toe
C. Irregular contour	Solar margin after resorption of fractures Subchondral bone with a displaced articular fracture
D. Combination destructive- productive change	Toe with osteomyelitis Solar area with osteomyelitis

This approach was necessary to provide information that incorporated fractures into the overall radiographic interpretation of the third phalanx. A more detailed discussion of the radiographic findings associated with third phalanx fractures is necessary to provide the AEP the background to more correctly interpret fractures of the third phalanx.

2. Classification of Third Phalanx Fractures

Fractures of P3 are classified into seven types based on the relationship with the distal interphalangeal joint (articular or non-articular), location (heel, extensor process, or solar margin), and plane of the fracture (non-sagittal or sagittal). This classification system, dependent on the radiographic interpretation, is typed in the following way:

Type I: Non-articular, heel
Type II: Articular, non-sagittal
Type III: Articular, sagittal
Type IV: Extensor process
Type V: Comminuted, secondary to foreign body penetration or osteomyelitis of only the body
Type VI: Non-articular, solar margin
Type VII: Palmar process in the foal

Type VI fractures are more common than the other five types combined. If the AEP is not identifying Type VI fractures in their practice, the reason is most likely their 65° DP-P3 radiographs are overexposed. An anecdotal story will emphasize this conclusion. At a national equine meeting, I presented a DEE of a horse with a history of foot lameness to a distal extremity "authority" for his interpretation. The radiographs were overexposed compromising his ability to evaluate the solar margin of P3, but they were of the quality this "authority" was accustomed to reviewing. An additional 65° DP-P3 taken with one-half the exposure time was later provided that clearly showed multiple solar margin fractures. The "authority" acknowledged the fractures but indicated those were "California Lesions" and not seen in the rest of the United States where horses did not live on concrete. Within six weeks of this meeting and following reduction of his exposure time for 65° DP-P3 by a factor of four, the "authority" telephoned to inform me he had diagnosed solar margin fractures as the cause of lameness in five horses. He was impressed but somewhat upset because he had not previously made this diagnosis in over 20 years.

3. Trabecular Pattern of the Body of the Third Phalanx

Interpretation must include a careful assessment of the trabecular pattern of P3 when solar margin fractures are identified. If there is increased coarseness of the trabecular pattern indicating an osteopenia, the solar margin fractures are usually pathologic fractures often secondary to laminitis. In addition, the fractures vary in size and number when associated with laminitis tending to be large, extensive, and multiple. Solar margin fractures with normal trabecular pattern to P3 tend to be small, focal, and single as well as associated with a more acute lameness of a moderate degree of severity.

4. Fracture or Packing Artifact

Both an acute Type II or III fracture and packing artifact can appear radiographically as a linear lucent finding. The differentiation between a fracture and packing artifact can be difficult, but there are three factors to be included in the interpretation to assist in this differentiation.
A. Clinical signs – the fracture will usually be associated with a severe degree of lameness.
B. The fracture will extend to and end at the margins of the third phalanx. The packing artifact may extend beyond the margins of P3.
C. Linear lucent packing artifacts are usually formed by gas in the medial and lateral sulci of the frog. These artifacts will be seen extending obliquely from the heel (abaxially) toward the toe (axially).

The Type II fractures run obliquely from the solar margin of the quarter (abaxially) towards the articulation (axially), and the Type III fracture runs sagittally from the toe to articulation.

If these factors do not allow the AEP to differentiate the linear lucency as either an artifact or fracture, the AEP has the options of repacking the foot and repeating the radiograph (usually the 65°DP-P3) or taking special projections, i.e., the D0°Pr-PaDiO and the heel view that highlights the area in question. It is recommended that repacking be done even if option two, i.e., special projections, is taken.

Type II and Type III fractures appear as a sharply marginated lucent line in the acute phase (Figure 6-16A). The fracture at the solar margin of P3 often can be identified as a single point of lucency with two linear lucencies of unequal width extending toward the distal interphalangeal joint. The narrower linear lucency represents the fracture line at the solar surface and the wider lucent line is located more dorsally. This difference in width is primarily a result of magnification, i.e., the solar surface is closer to the cassette when the exposure was made. Type II and III fractures will appear wider and more poorly marginated in the chronic phases. It is important to emphasize that assessment for healing of a Type II fracture may be difficult on the 65°DP-P3 so an oblique heel view is indicated (Figures 6-16 B and C).

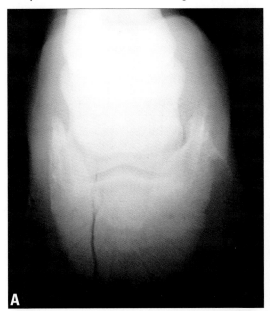

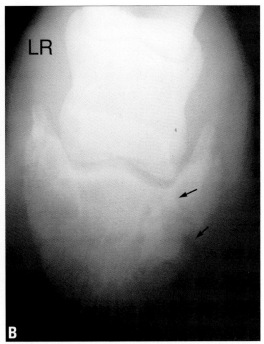

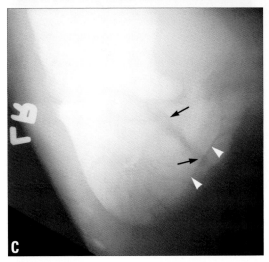

*Figure 6-16. An acute third phalanx fracture (Type III) will appear as a sharply marginated linear lucency within the margins of P3 (**A**). Chronic fractures (**B**) will appear wider and as a poorly marginated linear lucency (arrows). The oblique heel view (**C**) of B demonstrates the value of this special view for more accurately evaluating the degree of bone healing in this chronic Type II fracture. The linear shadow (arrowheads) running from the heel region towards the toe is created by a packing artifact.*

5. Palmar Process Fractures in the Foal

Ossicles of the medial and/or lateral palmar and plantar processes of P3 are seen in foals from a few weeks to a year in age. These ossicles are fractures (Type VII) rather than secondary centers of ossification or developmental orthopedic disease (DOD). These fractures may be seen in the club-footed foal and foals with or without clinical signs of lameness. The two radiographic patterns associated with this type of fracture are:

- A triangular bony fragment at the palmar aspect of the distal angle of the palmar process (Figure 6-17B).
- An oblong fragment separated from P3 by a lucent line extending 1-3 cm from the incisure of the palmar process to the solar margin (Figure 6-17C).

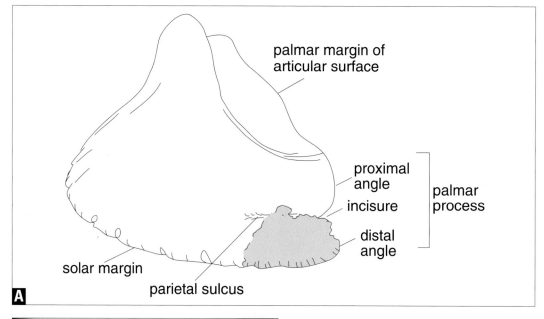

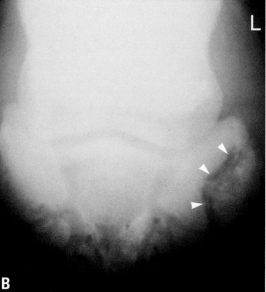

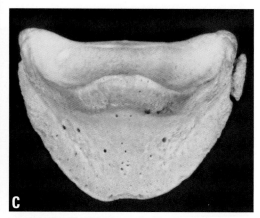

Figure 6-17. *The palmar process consists of a proximal and distal angle separated by the incisure (**A**). Palmar process fractures (arrowheads) in the foal are identified radiographically as either a triangular dense body at the palmar aspect of the distal angle of the palmar process (**B**) or as a separated oblong fragment involving the distal angle of the palmar process (**C**).*

These fractures are considered to result from unequal forces created by tension forces from the insertion of the deep digital flexor tendon on the solar surface and the compressive forces of weight bearing on the solar margin. These forces are concentrated in the region of the parietal sulcus which is thought to contribute to the development of these lesions (Figure 6-18).

Radiographic evidence of healing is commonly seen within 8-12 weeks. There does not seem to be significant long-term clinical consequences associated with these fractures and the club-footedness tends to be transient with proper management.

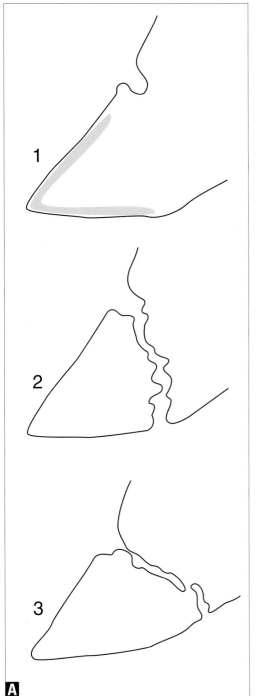

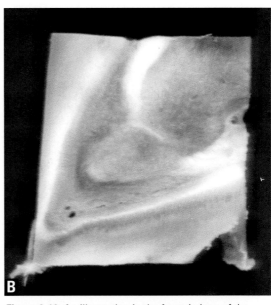

Figure 6-18. An illustration in the frontal plane of the region of the palmar process **(A)** demonstrates the normal appearance (1) of this area where the parietal sulcus is seen as an indentation in the dorsal cortical surface and the trabeculae are more parallel at the dorsal and solar cortices. A lucent line with a dense body seen radiographically results from disruption of the trabecular pattern extending from the area of the parietal sulcus to the solar cortex (2). Healing of a palmar process fracture usually has begun in 8-12 weeks (3) which is demonstrated in a pathologic specimen **(B)**.

NOTES

NOTES

NOTES

Chapter 7

Radiographic Interpretation of the Navicular Bone

I. Which Radiographic Views of the DEE are Important for Evaluation of the Navicular Bone?

II. Radiographic Anatomy of the Navicular Bone

III. Identification of Structural Changes in the Navicular Bone with the DEE
    1. LM View
    2. 65°DP Conedown View
    3. 45°DP View
    4. Flexor Skyline View
        A. Flexor Surface
        B. Flexor Cortex
        C. Medullary Cavity

IV. Identification of Structural Changes in the Navicular Bone using the Heel Projection

V. Navicular Disease
    1. Radiographic Signs of Degeneration of the Navicular Bone without Clinical Signs
    2. Clinical Signs of Degeneration of the Navicular Bone without Radiographic Signs

VI. Conclusions

I. Which Radiographic Views of the DEE are Important for the Evaluation of the Navicular Bone?

The radiographic evaluation of the navicular bone is accomplished primarily using the 65°DP conedown, the 45°DP, and the flexor skyline projections. The LM view provides diagnostic information that tends to be supplemental to these other three views. The 65°DP-P3 does not contribute to interpretation of the navicular bone because the navicular bone cannot be visualized on this view. The dorso65°proximo45°lateral (medial)-palmarodistomedial (lateral) oblique (the heel projection) is a special view that provides valuable information concerning the extremity and distal abaxial region of the navicular bone.

There will be times when a complete radiographic examination cannot be obtained. A view, e.g., the flexor skyline, may not be possible to obtain because the horse, even with sedation, cannot be positioned correctly without possible bodily harm or destruction of your equipment. It is important that the reason(s) for not obtaining a complete DEE be noted in the medical record to prevent potential charges of negligence.

II. Radiographic Anatomy of the Navicular Bone

The normal navicular bone seen on the LM is essentially rectangular in shape with the proximodistal dimension slightly greater than the dorsopalmar (Figure 7-1). It is described as having two borders (proximal and distal) and two surfaces (articular and flexor). The navicular bone is fixed by a suspensory apparatus which includes the medial and lateral navicular suspensory ligaments extending obliquely from the dorsal abaxial surface of distal P1 to the

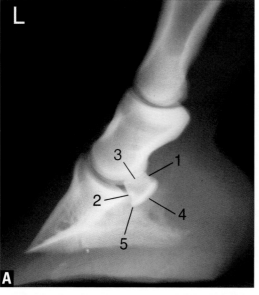 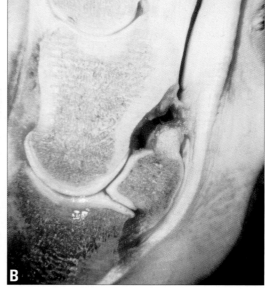

Figure 7-1. The LM radiographic view **(A)** permits the proximal (1) and distal (2) borders and the articular (3) and flexor (4) surfaces of the navicular to be evaluated. The flexor cortex and the distal extension of the flexor cortex (5) or distal flexor border (DFB) must be evaluated on the LM view. A specimen **(B)** shows the navicular bone and its suspensory apparatus in cross-section.

proximal border of the navicular bone. The impar or distal suspensory ligament of the navicular bone extends from the distal border of the navicular bone to the flexor surface of P3 at midline. The deep digital flexor tendon runs over the flexor surface of the navicular bone to the flexor surface of P3 attaching into the semilunar crest. This attachment is distal to that of the impar ligament and extends more abaxially (Figure 7-2).

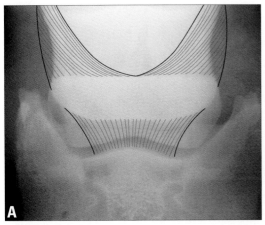
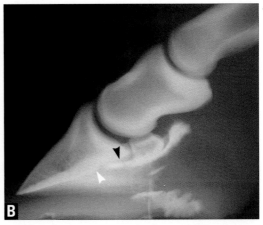

Figure 7-2. *Productive structural changes seen on the LM view occur at the sites of attachment of the suspensory apparatus of the navicular bone. The medial and lateral suspensory ligaments originate from the dorsoabaxial surface of distal P1 and insert on the extremities and proximal border of the navicular bone . The distal part of the suspensory apparatus of the navicular bone is the impar or distal suspensory ligament of the navicular bone which originates from the distal border and inserts near midline on the flexor surface of P3 (A). The deep digital flexor (DDF) tendon runs over the flexor surface of the navicular bone inserting at the semilunar crest of P3 more distally and over a larger area than the impar ligament. Contrast placed within the navicular bursa (B) demonstrates the attachments of the impar ligament in the area dorsal to the contrast (black arrowhead) and the DDF tendon in the area palmarodistal to the contrast (white arrowhead). These attachments near midline are seen in Figure 7-1B.*

The navicular bone has a distinct medullary cavity, flexor cortex, flexor cortical surface, and extremities. These anatomical areas can be seen collectively on the flexor skyline view (Figure 7-3). The trabecular pattern of the medullary cavity is seen dorsal to the dense flexor cortex. The end-on vascular canals can be identified as circular lucencies in the medullary cavity. The flexor cortex with a distinct interface with the medullary cavity is evident in the normal navicular bone, and the central protuberance projecting palmarly is called the "navicular ridge." The flexor surface appears as a smooth contour and the medial and lateral extremities are rounded.

Figure 7-3. *The central palmar protuberance of the flexor cortex is the "navicular ridge" (1). The flexor skyline view (extended Pa50°Pr-PaDiO) allows the anatomical features of the flexor cortical surface (2), flexor cortex (3), the medullary cavity (4), and extremities (5) to be evaluated. The trabecular pattern of the medullary cavity and dense flexor cortex form a sharp interface in the navicular bone without chronic remodeling changes.*

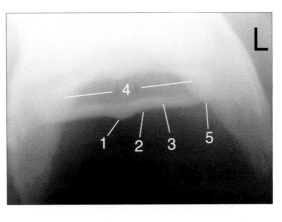

Important anatomical areas seen on the 65°DP conedown (D65°Pr-PaDiO) are the distal flexor border (DFB) and distal body of the navicular bone as well as the subchondral bone of the distal interphalangeal joint (Figure 7-4). Interpretation of the DFB is extremely important, but the AEP tends to misdiagnose changes in the DFB for two reasons. The first is a technical problem: The angulation in the proximal direction must be great enough to superimpose the image of the DFB on mid-P2 and the

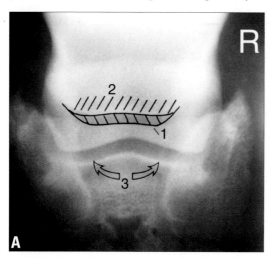
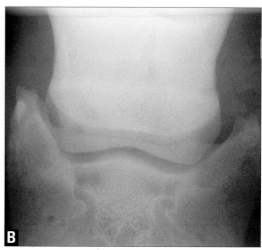

Figure 7-4. *The DFB (1) and distal body (2) of the navicular bone and the subchondral bone of the distal interphalangeal joint (3) are anatomical areas best evaluated on the 65°DP conedown (**A**). It is extremely important that the radiographic quality of this view permits the DFB to be evaluated. A well-positioned 65° DP conedown (**B**) allows evaluation of these 3 areas.*

exposure must permit detailed bony evaluation without preparation artifacts. The second is a knowledge problem. The DFB appears as a uniform bony density with a straight contour projecting distal to the distal border. The DFB can be seen on the LM as a "lip" of bone at the distal flexor surface (see Figure 7-1).

The body of the navicular bone can be evaluated on both the 65°DP conedown and the 45°DP views. The distal body (one half) should be evaluated primarily on the 65°DP conedown and the proximal body (one half), proximal border, and extremities should be evaluated primarily using the 45°DP (Figure 7-5). Both views are valuable in evaluating potential change(s) in the central one-third of the body of the navicular bone.

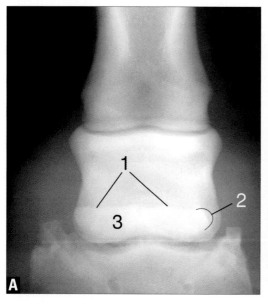
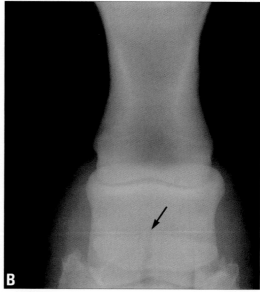

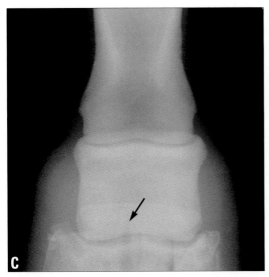
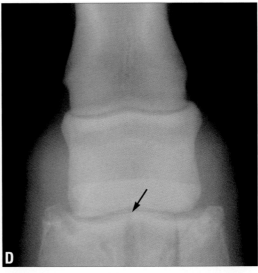

Figure 7-5. The proximal border (1), both extremities (2), and the proximal body (3) are anatomical areas best evaluated *(A)* on the 45°DP (D45°Pr-PaDiO). The importance of 45° proximal angulation *(B)* in evaluating the proximal body of the navicular bone is demonstrated by comparing it to a 37° *(C)* and 30° *(D)* proximal angulation. The position of the proximal extent of the central sulcus packing artifact (arrow) can be correlated to the degree of angulation.

III. Identification of Structural Changes in the Navicular Bone using the DEE

The AEP must interpret radiographic changes in the navicular bone using each view of the DEE before establishing "Conclusions and Impressions." **Always remember…a one-view radiographic examination is no radiographic examination!** Therefore, the radiographic changes and their locations will be correlated to each radiographic view. A comparison of the central body on both the 45°DP and the 65°DP conedown is important in the differentiation of a navicular lesion from an artifact (Figure 7-6). However, the 65°DP conedown should not be used to evaluate changes at the

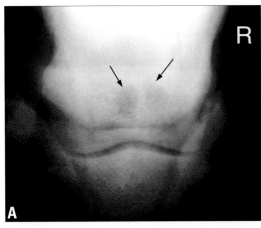
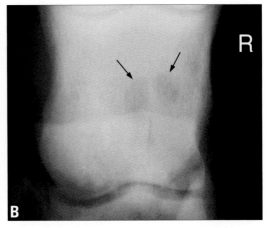

Figure 7-6. Interpretation of a radiographic finding seen on one view must include its evaluation of all views of the DEE. The two lucencies (arrows) seen in the mid-body of the navicular bone with the 65°DP conedown *(A)* must be correlated with the findings seen on the 45°DP *(B)*. In this example, the lucencies are not within the body of the navicular bone. What should be the next step in the radiographic evaluation? (Hint: Reread the first sentence.)

proximal border and extremities because magnification makes productive changes in these areas appear larger and distorted. It must be emphasized that the location(s) of change(s) identified or suspected must be correlated to the similar anatomical location on different views (Figure 7-7).

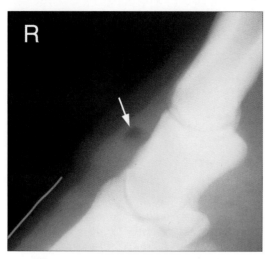

Figure 7-7. The location of change(s) identified or suspected must be evaluated on all the views of the DEE. An evaluation of the LM view revealed that the two lucencies in Figure 7-6 are artifacts produced by iatrogenic gas dorsal to the second phalanx.

1. LM View
Productive Changes
The radiographic signs of navicular bone pathology seen on the LM are bony production, density, and contour changes. The productive bony change is seen on both the proximal and distal borders with the former location much more common and extensive. Productive bony change will result in the radiographic appearance of the navicular bone changing shape from rectangular to oblong (Figure 7-8). The bone overall appears more dense and there is a loss of the trabecular pattern. The 45°DP will confirm the productive change on the proximal border and extremities. On the flexor skyline view, the navicular bone will appear more dense with an apparent loss of the trabecular pattern of the medullary cavity created by the productive bone on the borders. The extremities on the skyline view will lose the normal rounded appearance and become angulated. These changes in shape and density of the navicular bone are primarily caused by remodeling at the attachment of the suspensory ligaments of the navicular bone (enthesophytes).

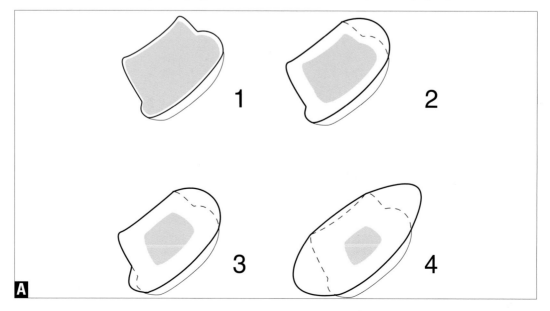

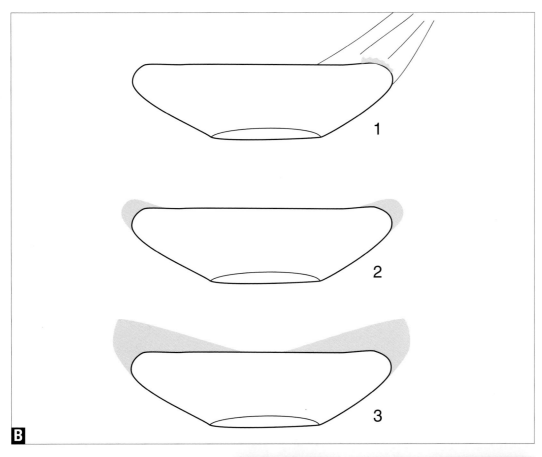

B

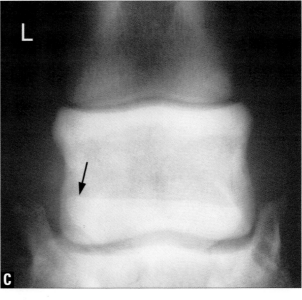

L

C

Figure 7-8. Productive bony change (2-4) in the suspensory ligaments of the navicular bone both proximally and distally results in a change in shape and elongation of the normal (1) navicular bone on the LM *(A)*. This change is seen on the 45°DP as a change in shape at the proximal border *(B)* which can involve one *(C)* or both extremities. The change in shape of the one extremity (arrow) seen on this radiograph is not positional because the proximal and distal interphalangeal joint spaces are parallel. The proximal border of the normal navicular bone should also be parallel with these joint spaces (see Figure 7-5 A).

Density Changes

Focal density changes on the LM view include areas of increased and decreased density. Increased density may be seen in the tissues distal to the distal border (avulsion fracture) and proximal to the proximal border (calcification in the medial and/or lateral navicular suspensory ligaments or fracture of these enthesophytes) of the navicular bone (Figure 7-9). Soft tissue mineralization in the palmar heel region may also be identified on the LM view, but the flexor skyline view is required to localize this density. Multiple corticosteroid injections into the navicular bursal region can result in dystrophic calcification of the deep digital flexor tendon and digital cushion. Degeneration of the navicular bone is a common underlying disorder seen radiographically.

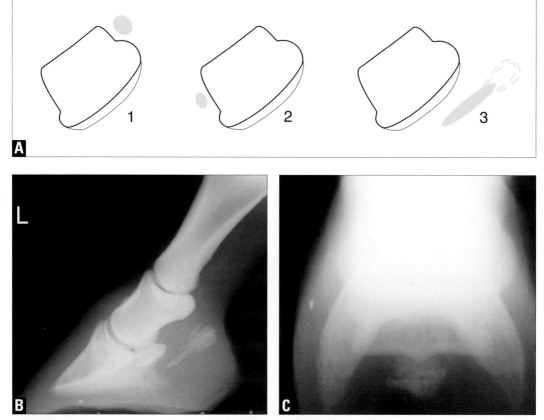

Figure 7-9. *Focal increased densities can be identified on the LM view at both borders of the navicular bone and palmarly* ***(A)***. *A discrete focal density proximal to the proximal border (1) can result from dystrophic calcification or a fracture. A poorly marginated density distal to the distal border (2) is more commonly seen and represents an avulsion fracture. Calcification of the soft tissues in the heel region can be seen palmar to the navicular bone (3). A severe degree of palmar soft tissue mineralization seen on the LM* ***(B)*** *and skyline views* ***(C)*** *is usually associated with a history of multiple corticosteroid injections into the heel region.*

An increased focal density distal to the navicular bone should be evaluated on the 65°DP conedown and flexor skyline, but the special heel view (D65°Pr45°M[L]-PaDiL[M]O) may be required for precise localization. The increased focal density proximally requires evaluation of the 45°DP rather than the 65°DP conedown, but the flexor skyline and heel views (D65°Pr45°M(L)-PaDiL(M)O) are beneficial for a complete assessment and often allow one to change a "suspected" lesion to a "confirmed" lesion.

Contour Change

A focal lucent change of the navicular bone is often identified with a contour change. These findings are seen on the LM in two locations: the midpoints of the flexor cortex and the distal border (Figure 7-10). These lucencies are commonly associated with degeneration. However, the lucency involving the mid-region of the distal flexor border occurs secondary to synovial invagination and that in the flexor cortex may also be a remodeling change.

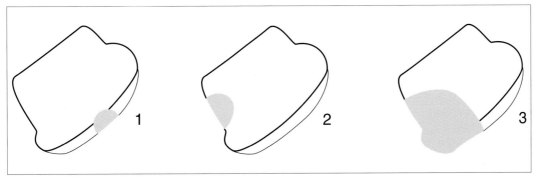

Figure 7-10. *Lucent change in the navicular bone seen on the LM view occurs in conjunction with a contour change in the midpoints of the flexor cortex (1) and distal border (2). Chronic degeneration can result in a more lucent appearance to the distal body of the navicular bone (3).*

2. The 65°DP Conedown View

The radiographic signs of navicular bone pathology seen on the 65°DP conedown are bony destruction, density, and contour changes. Destructive and density (lucency) changes are commonly seen together when evaluating the distal body and DFB. This is a pathological result of hyperemia which stimulates osteoclastic and synovial activity. The result is a loss of bone and an increase in synovial tissue extending into the area seen radiographically as lucent areas. The lucencies can vary in shape from linear to cystic, and the cystic area(s) can be isolated or coalescing (Figure 7-11). Linear lucencies can be a result of packing artifacts, vascular canals, or fractures. The vascular canals are differentiated from fractures because they are multiple, have a foramen at the distal border, appear less lucent than a fracture, and cannot be seen extending into the proximal one-half of the body of the navicular bone. Remodeling at the vascular foramen and widening of the canals produces an inverted "V"-shaped appearance. An interesting correlation can be made between the similarities in the radiographic findings in the navicular (distal sesamoid) bone and the findings described for sesamoiditis of the proximal sesamoid bones (see p.156).

Contour change on the 65°DP conedown occurs at the DFB and at the angle of the distal body of the navicular bone. An irregularity of the DFB results from bony resorption (Figure 7-12). Commonly this DFB contour irregularity accompanies cystic lucencies in the distal body of the navicular bone and is a sign of degeneration. DFB irregularity tends to result in secondary pathology in the deep digital flexor tendon and there tends to be a high degree of correlation between this irregularity and clinical lameness.

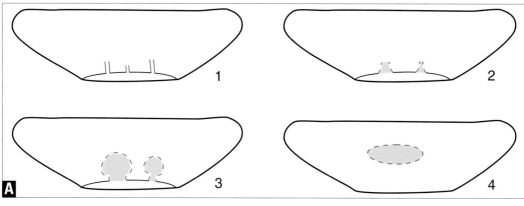

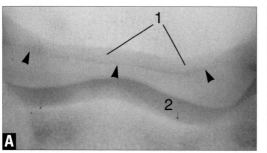

Figure 7-11. *Lucencies seen in the navicular bone on the 65°DP conedown can vary from linear to cystic with the cystic change being solitary or multiple (A). Linear lucencies with a distinct foramen and parallel walls are normal nutrient foramina and canals (1). Resorption at the foramen at the distal border and widening of the vascular canal (2) are early remodeling changes. Cystic lucencies (3) are indicative of degeneration and can be isolated (4) or coalescing (B).*

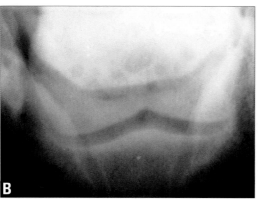

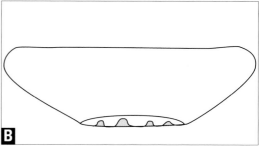

Figure 7-12. *The DFB (1) must be visible on the 65° DP conedown proximal to the joint space (2) and palmar border (arrowheads) of proximal P3 (A). Irregularity to the silhouette of the DFB correlates closely with clinical signs of lameness (B).*

The contour change at the angle of the distal body of the navicular bone is commonly associated with a fracture. These fractures may be either unilateral or bilateral and involve the medial and/or lateral aspects of the navicular bone. It is important to realize that this contour change can be associated with a focal lucent defect with or without evidence of a fracture fragment (Figure 7-13). The fracture fragment may not be visible with chronic fractures because of resorption. These fractures are avulsion-type and retain a blood supply via the impar ligament allowing resorption. Another radiographic determination is the overall condition of the distal body compatible with degeneration. Avulsion fractures can be seen associated with or without normal trabecular pattern and flexor cortical density. A fracture with a normal appearing trabecular pattern tends to produce a transient lameness of a mild to moderate degree lasting for a few days and the prognosis for clinical soundness is much better than with degenerate bone where it is a pathologic fracture (Figure 7-14). Finally, it is important to realize these fractures are commonly seen in the high performance horse.

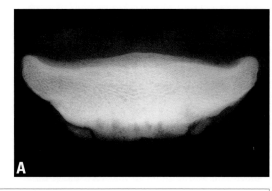

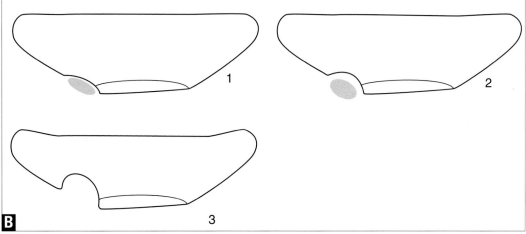

Figure 7-13. *Avulsion fractures from the distal flexor border occur at specific locations and appear as a separate dense body with contour change as demonstrated in this specimen **(A)**. The fracture fragment (1) can undergo partial (2) or total (3) resorption but the lucent contour change of the fracture site remains identifiable **(B)**.*

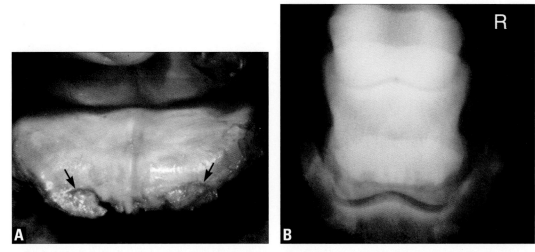

Figure 7-14. *Avulsion fractures occur with **(A)** and without evidence of degeneration of the navicular bone. Note the fractures (arrows) are on both sides of the navicular bone, and the distal flexor border is irregular as illustrated in Figure 7-12B. The positioning of the radiographic view **(B)** is less than 65° proximal so the DFB is difficult to evaluate because it is superimposed on the palmar border of proximal P3. Fractures without radiographic evidence of degeneration may be unilateral or bilateral as well as medial and/or lateral and the prognosis for performance soundness tends to be much better when there is an absence of radiographic signs of degeneration.*

3. The 45°DP View

The 45°DP view is important for evaluating the proximal border, extremities, and proximal one-half of the body of the navicular bone. The radiographic signs identified on this view are bony production and density changes. The density change is seen as linear or cystic lucencies in the body of the navicular bone and must be correlated to similar findings on the 65°DP conedown.

Productive bony change is seen on the proximal border and extremities of the navicular bone in the areas of attachment of the medial and/or lateral navicular suspensory ligament. This change on the 45°DP view should be correlated to similar change on the LM view for more complete interpretation. It is important to realize this finding indicates chronic remodeling resulting from injury. The acute injury to the fibro-osseous interface of the ligament and navicular bone is a tearing of ligamentous fibers and subsequent hemorrhage (see Figure 7-8 B1). There will not be radiographic signs that can be correlated to clinical signs associated with this acute injury.

Density change seen on the 45°DP is commonly a lucency located in the body of the navicular bone. These lucencies represent either pathologic change (degeneration) or artifact. Both can appear linear or cystic.

Artifactual linear lucencies seen on the 45°DP must be differentiated from fractures. Artifactual linear lucencies are commonly seen and result from improper packing of the sulci of the frog. The collateral sulcus artifact is seen superimposed on the image of the navicular bone and it runs obliquely from the heel toward midline while the central sulcus of the frog artifact runs saggitally near midline. The length of the sulci artifacts superimposed on the image of the navicular bone is variable. **A diagnostic key for a fracture** is that the linear lucency must be within the silhouette of the bone. Therefore, a linear lucency comparison using both the 45°DP and 65°DP conedown usually reveals the artifactual lucency extends beyond the margins of the navicular bone on one or both views. The differentiation of an artifactual linear lucency is completed by an evaluation of the flexor skyline view using the same principle (Figure 7-15).

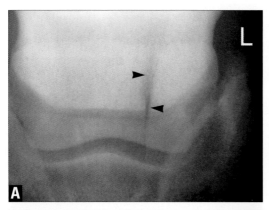

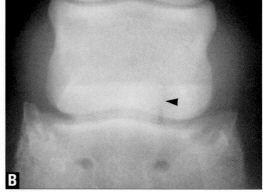

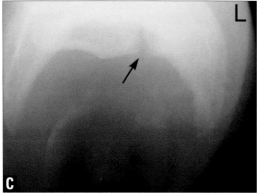

Figure 7-15. Interpret all radiographic views to confirm a suspected lesion. A linear lucency (arrowheads) is seen on the 65°DP conedown *(A)* superimposed on the lateral wing of the navicular bone, but the lucency extends beyond the borders of the navicular bone and appears to be a packing artifact. A linear lucency (arrowhead) is seen in the proximal body of the navicular bone on the 45°DP *(B)* but a processing artifact is seen. The "suspected" fracture is confirmed on the flexor skyline view *(C)* by the change in contour at the flexor surface (arrow) and a poorly defined linear lucency in the flexor cortex that extends through the medullary cavity.

Cystic lucencies in the body of the navicular bone are commonly identified on the 45°DP. The cystic lesions are not associated with the proximal border or extremities. The lucent change may be confined to a focal location in the navicular bone near midline or be extensive in the medial to lateral dimension. These patterns of distribution are compatible with degeneration and must be evaluated on the 65° conedown and the flexor skyline views for completeness.

4. The Flexor Skyline View (Extended Pa50°Pr-PaDiO)

The flexor skyline view is very important for a complete radiographic evaluation of the morphology of the navicular bone. This view is extremely valuable for interpreting changes to the medullary cavity, flexor cortex, flexor surface, and the soft tissues palmar to the navicular bone. The radiographic changes seen relate to the anatomical area where these changes occur. In general, the radiographic changes are density, contour, productive, and destructive.

A. Flexor Surface

The change seen at the flexor surface on the skyline view is in the contour. Abnormal contour results from a destructive change extending from the cortex or from the soft tissues associated with a penetrating wound (Figure 7-16). The 65°DP conedown is the primary comparison view for complete evaluation of a contour change at the flexor surface with destruction of the underlying flexor cortex. If a productive change accompanies the flexor surface contour change, it occurs at the extremities of the navicular bone. The 45°DP is the primary view for a complete evaluation of these changes.

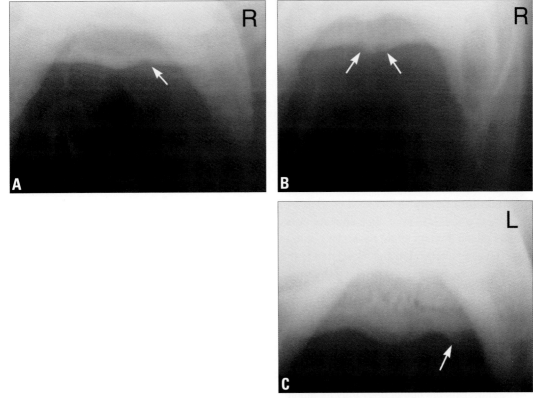

Figure 7-16. *A penetrating wound into the sole can extend to the flexor surface producing a focal abnormal contour at the flexor surface due to destruction **(A)**. An irregular flexor surface to the navicular bone extending over a few millimeters to centimeters can be a result of destruction created by either an infection in the navicular bursa with osteomyelitis or degeneration **(B)**. The history and clinical signs permit differentiation of infection and degeneration. A productive change at the flexor surface (arrow) is an uncommon finding but when identified it tends to be near the lateral extremity of a navicular bone **(C)**.*

B. Flexor Cortex

Flexor cortex abnormalities are identified by density change. The density change in the flexor cortex tends to be a lucency that is either cystic or linear resulting in a loss of the continuity of the stripe of the dense bone. The most common cause of flexor cortex lucency is degeneration of the navicular bone, but osteomyelitis will also produce this change. Osteomyelitis may be differentiated by the clinical history and examination, but differentiation on radiographic signs is based on identifying a productive response surrounding the cortical lucency (Figure 7-17). As indicated previously, a linear lucency produced by a fracture line or packing artifact can usually be differentiated using the flexor skyline view.

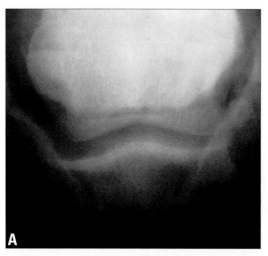
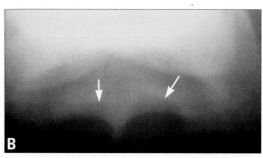

Figure 7-17. *An unsuccessfully treated osteomyelitis of the navicular bone secondary to a penetrating wound can produce extensive cortical and medullary bony destruction* **(A)**. *This lesion, unlike degeneration, will also have a productive change (arrows) surrounding the lucency seen best on the skyline view* **(B)**.

C. Medullary Cavity

The loss of trabeculation of the medullary cavity on the flexor skyline view is a result of productive change on the borders of the navicular bone, especially the proximal border. The 45°DP and LM views must be interpreted and correlated to this finding on the flexor skyline. The experience of the author indicates that the productive change on the borders creates this radiographic appearance rather than an actual sclerosis within the medullary cavity.

The evaluation of the medullary cavity should confirm the presence of avulsion fractures from the distal body of the navicular bone and a sharp cortico-medullary junction. These fractures are identified in a specific location as a dense body that is poorly marginated and the density may be medially, laterally, or both (Figure 7-18). When there is a significant degree of bone destruction at the fracture site, the dense body may be highlighted by a zone of lucency. This occurs more commonly when there is a significant degree of degeneration and the fracture is pathological. The loss of the distinct cortico-medullary junction is associated with degeneration of the navicular bone but this finding must not be considered pathognomic for degeneration.

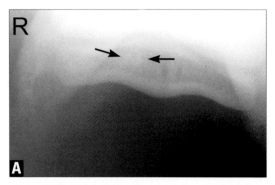
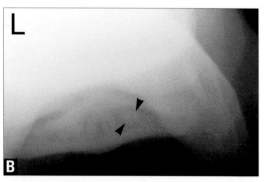

Figure 7-18. The avulsion fracture from the distal flexor border can be identified on the flexor skyline view as a poorly marginated density (arrows) superimposed on the medullary cavity at a specific location *(A)*. The dense body appears highlighted (arrowheads) when extensive destruction has occurred in the distal body of the navicular bone at the fracture site *(B)*.

IV. Identification of Structural Changes in the Navicular Bone using a Special View: Heel Projection [Dorso65°Proximo45°Medial (Lateral) – PalmaroDistoLateral(Medial) Oblique]

A special radiographic view is taken to supplement the routine DEE for examination of the navicular bone. This view is taken 45° from the mid-sagittal plane and permits evaluation of the extremity and abaxial region of the distal body of the navicular bone. The radiographic signs identified are density and contour changes.

The extremity of the navicular bone is a region where packing artifacts and fractures are commonly seen as linear lucencies. Productive change produces an abnormal contour to the extremity and the heel view provides radiographic information to supplement findings seen or suspected on the 45°DP, flexor skyline, and LM views.

The abaxial region of the distal body is a common site for avulsion fractures. The avulsion fracture fragment may better be identified on the heel view than routine views. The site of origin of the fracture appears as a density and contour change. A lucent defect in this specific area is compatible with a site of a fracture even though the fracture fragment may not be seen. As discussed previously, the fracture fragment may have resorbed or it may be a pathological fracture associated with degeneration of the navicular bone. The radiographic evaluation of the distal body of the navicular bone for signs of degeneration is an important radiographic determination because a pathologic fracture has a significantly poorer prognosis for soundness (Figure 7-19).

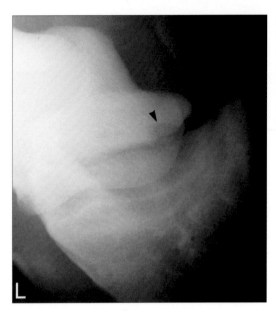

Figure 7-19. *Avulsion fractures from the distal abaxial region of the navicular bone can be more completely evaluated using an oblique heel projection (D65°Pr45°M(L) – PaDiL(M)O). The special view for the highlighted lesion seen in Figure 7-18 B demonstrates the value of this special projection, where a large lucency (arrowhead) at the site of origin of the faintly visualized fracture can be seen.*

V. Navicular Disease

The role of radiology in the diagnosis of navicular disease (ND) is major and controversial. The controversy is in part a result of the complex etiology and the progressive nature of the disease process.

The complex etiology is a result of uncertainty of the precise cause(s) of this disease. Conformation and genetic factors are involved and the alteration of blood flow leading to remodeling is directly associated with the radiographic signs of this disease process. This disease process is a degenerative process that is progressive. The rate of progression tends to be variable.

ND is considered by many AEP to be a clinical diagnosis rather than a radiographic diagnosis. Part of the explanation for this consideration may be a lack of understanding of the radiographic findings.

The radiographic signs of ND are density and contour changes in the distal body, flexor cortex, and DFB. The density change is seen radiographically as lucencies which result from destruction associated with increased vascularity and osteoclastic activity.

The locations of lucent changes are restricted to the body, flexor cortex, and DFB in the palmaro-distal region of the navicular bone (Figure 7-20). Radiographic signs of ND are not identified at the proximal border and adjacent body of the navicular bone. Lucencies in the body of the navicular bone seen on the 65°DP conedown vary in shape from straight to cystic, in number from single to multiple, and in diameter from a millimeter to centimeter in diameter. The lucency when created by normal vascular canals tends to be straight walled, few (three or four) in number, and less than two millimeters in diameter. The foramen associated with vascular canals tends to have distinct, sharp margins. There is a wide variation in the shape, size, and number of lucencies associated with ND which are indicative of the degree of remodeling. This remodeling is dynamic and progressive. It is identified initially as loss of the vascular foramen and widened lucencies in the distal body that tend to become bulbous and cystic in shape. The number of lucencies can be

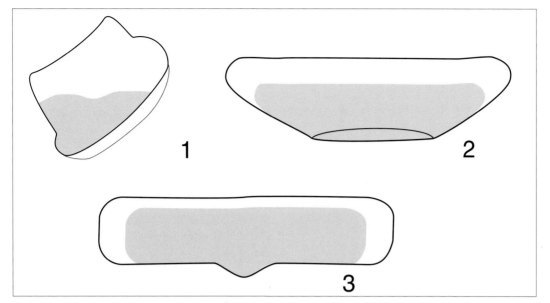

Figure 7-20. The radiographic changes seen with navicular bone degeneration are schematically located in the palmarodistal region (shaded area) of the navicular bone on the LM view (1). These changes are correlated to areas identified on the 65°DP conedown (2) and the flexor skyline (3) views. Note that degeneration of the navicular bone does not involve the proximal border or the articular surface of the navicular bone.

single but more commonly tends to be multiple. The lucencies tend to be more poorly marginated when seen in multiples versus more sharply marginated when single and large. On the flexor skyline view, these lucencies are seen in the medullary cavity and are associated with loss of the flexor cortex. An early sign of flexor cortical disease is a loss of the sharply defined corticomedullary junction in a focal location. Lucency of the flexor cortex is compatible with destruction and can lead to breakdown of the subchondral bone at the flexor surface (Figure 7-21). Granulation tissue extends onto the flexor surface and progresses abaxially resulting in loss of nutrition to the fibrocartilage of the flexor surface. Secondary change in the navicular bursa, deep digital flexor tendon, and flexor cortical bone follows.

The correlation of clinical and radiographic findings tends to cause great difficulty for many AEP. This correlation is worthy of discussion so a radiologist's perception will be provided to supplement the much stronger background the AEP has for evaluating clinical signs.

As a starting point, the radiographic interpretation of the navicular bone for structural changes should **always** be done independent of the clinical signs. Always **follow** with a correlation of clinical and radiographic signs. This technique avoids neglecting and leaving out important radiographic findings or committing the error of omission which is very common in equine radiology.

There are many patients where the clinical and radiographic signs are compatible. These are not the patients requiring further discussion. Further discussion is important in those two groups of horses with a disparity between the clinical signs and radiographic findings.

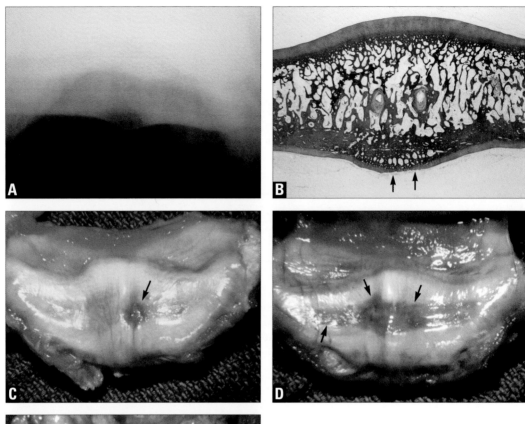

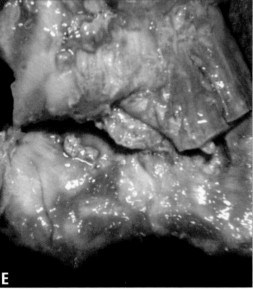

Figure 7-21. Lucency of the flexor cortex *(A)* is compatible with breakdown of the subchondral bone and fibrocartilage (arrows) at the flexor surface commonly at the navicular ridge *(B)*. This breakdown allows granulation tissue (arrow) to extend onto the flexor surface *(C)* and progress abaxially *(D)* resulting in a barrier which causes a loss of nutrition to the underlying fibrocartilage of the flexor surface. Secondary changes in the navicular bursa, deep flexor tendon, and underlying flexor cortical bone follow *(E)*. Adhesions and the development of a "mechanical" lameness can result.

1. Radiographic Signs of Degeneration of the Navicular Bone without Clinical Signs

This disparity does occur in routine examinations but it is most important when associated with purchase work. It is imperative that the radiographic changes be reported because radiographic evidence of degeneration can be seen **before** clinical signs are detected by the AEP. Some equine practitioners have difficulty in accepting this conclusion. Most veterinarians have been taught and should understand that there is **not** a direct correlation between the severity of clinical and radiographic signs of bone and joint disease.

To demonstrate this point, an orthopedic problem in the dog known to all veterinarians will be used, i.e., canine hip dysplasia. The coxofemoral joints of dogs are radiographed to qualify for breeding purposes. Radiographic evidence of shallow acetabula, subluxation of the coxofemoral joints, and a moderate degree of remodeling changes of the femoral heads and necks are radiographic findings observed in a two-year old German Shepherd dog. The owner and trainer insist the dog has never taken a lame step in its life, and the dog's veterinarian could not document a past or present lameness. None the less, this patient by definition has canine hip dysplasia. Radiographic evidence of degeneration or other radiographic change without clinical signs of lameness is evidence of bony damage in an individual horse that is fortunate enough not to be lame at that time. It is very important that the radiographic evidence of change be disclosed to the client and recorded in the medical record. Furthermore, it is clear, based on years of experience dealing with numerous horses, that one is unable to predict if or when an individual horse will experience lameness.

2. Clinical Signs of Navicular Disease without Radiographic Signs

This disparity is less common. It is important to remember that there are other causes of caudal heel syndrome that may be producing the clinical signs. These conditions must be excluded as the cause of the clinical signs before a clinical diagnosis of ND can be concluded. However, as a general conclusion, radiographic signs are commonly seen **after** there are signs of clinical disease. Associated with this disparity, nuclear scanning has been shown to provide important diagnostic information months prior to radiographic evidence of degeneration (Figure 7-22). If nuclear scanning is unavailable to the AEP, follow-up radiographic examinations in three to six months may document the clinical diagnosis of navicular disease.

The important issues for the AEP to realize are:
- **A disparity between clinical and radiographic signs of degeneration of the navicular bone exists.**
- **Radiographic evidence of navicular bone degeneration can be diagnostic.**
- **The clinical diagnosis of navicular disease without radiographic confirmation may be confirmed with nuclear imaging or follow-up radiographs at a later date.**

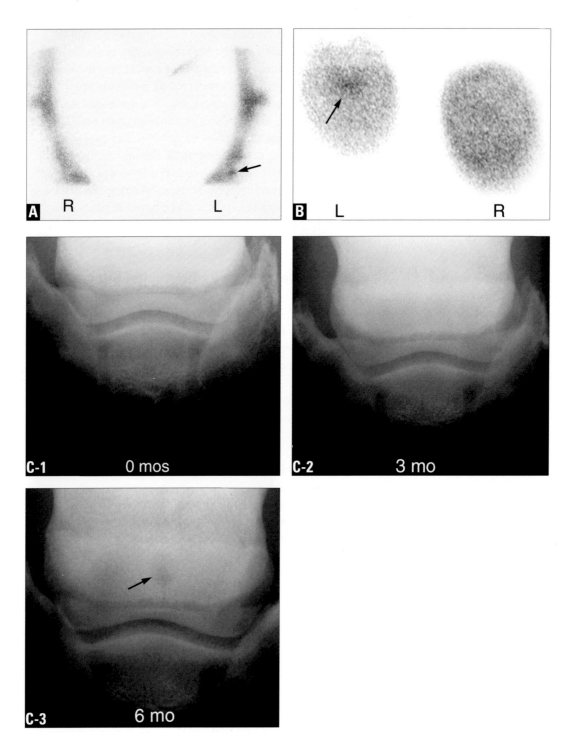

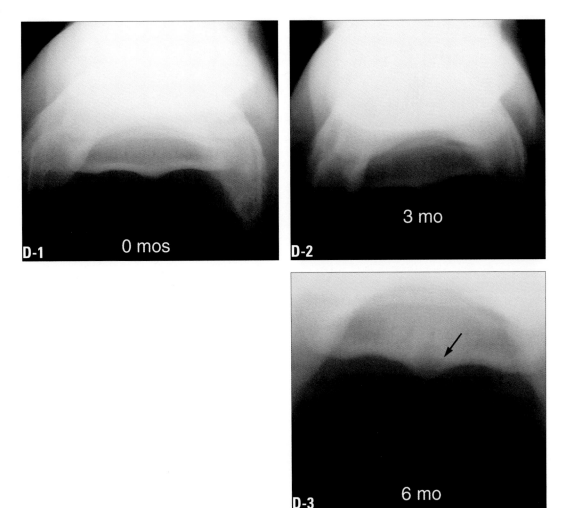

Figure 7-22. *A disparity in clinical and radiographic signs existed where there were clinical signs of left front navicular disease without radiographic changes. The LM **(A)** and palmar **(B)** nuclear scintigraphic images permitted resolution of this disparity months before radiographic signs could be identified. The 65°DP conedown **(C)** and flexor skyline **(D)** views at 0, 3, and 6 months demonstrate the development of radiographic evidence of degeneration (arrows) during a six-month period after a positive bone scan of the left front navicular bone.*

VI. Conclusions

Radiographic interpretation of the navicular bone is accomplished by a complete evaluation of the 65°DP conedown, the 45°DP, the flexor skyline, and the LM views. It is extremely important to know and follow this process and always remember... **"A one-view radiographic examination is no examination."***

*Note: This important radiographic principle can be reinforced by interpreting only the 65°DP conedown views shown in Figures 7-6A and 7-17A.

NOTES

NOTES

NOTES

NOTES

NOTES

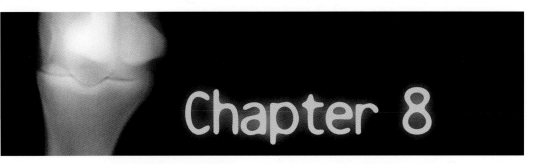

Chapter 8

Radiographic Interpretation of the Fetlock

I. Radiography of the Fetlock

1. Views of the Routine Radiographic Examination

A routine radiographic examination of the fetlock should consist of five projections. Three special projections are taken to evaluate the palmarodistal MC III, dorsodistal MCIII and the abaxial recess of the proximal sesamoid bone. The five routine views (Figures 8-1, 8-2, 8-3, 8-4, and 8-5) are:

1. Dorsopalmar (DP)
2. Lateromedial (LM)
3. Flexed lateromedial (F-LM)
4. Medial oblique (MO)
5. Lateral oblique (LO)

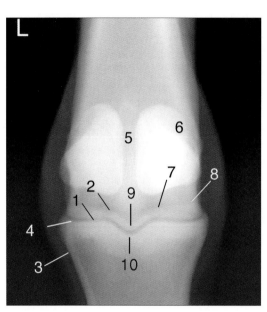

Figure 8-1. *The D30°Pr-PaDiO view allows evaluation of the joint space width (1), the trabecular bony detail of the subchondral bone of distal MCIII (2) and proximal P1, the medial and lateral periosteal surfaces (3), the periarticular margins of the joint (4), and the medial and lateral soft tissue thickness. The axial (5) and abaxial (6) regions of the proximal sesamoid should be evaluated for productive and destructive bony changes. The dorsal border of proximal P1 can be differentiated from the palmar border on the DP by the dorsal eminences (7) which are located near midline and slope abaxially while the palmar border is identified by the palmar eminences (8) which are more proximal abaxial and slope distally towards midline. Located at midline are the sagittal ridge (9) and the sagittal groove (10)*

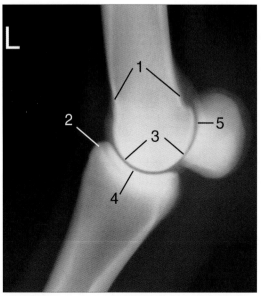

Figure 8-2. *The LM view permits evaluation of the joint capsule, the dorsal and palmar periarticular regions of distal MCIII (1) and proximal P1 (2), and the subchondral bone of the condyle of MCIII (3), proximal P1 (4) and the sesamoid bones (5). The dorsal and palmar periosteal surfaces and cortices of MCIII, P1 and P2 and, when included on the radiograph, the proximal and distal interphalangeal joints should also be interpreted.*

Figure 8-3. The flexed-lateromedial (f-LM) view permits interpretation of anatomical structures of the fetlock similar to the LM, but flexion permits better evaluation of the dorsal sagittal ridge, condylar surfaces and subchondral bone of distal MCIII and proximal P1 as well as the periarticular and articular surface of the proximal sesamoid bones.

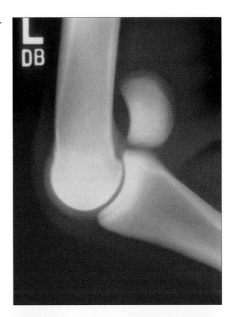

Figure 8-4. The D30°Pr60°L-PaDiMO view of the fetlock allows interpretation of the dorsomedial and palmarolateral contours of the fetlock. The medial dorsal eminence (arrow) is best evaluated for fractures using this view.

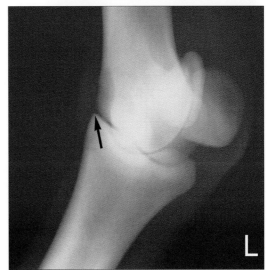

Figure 8-5. The D30°Pr60°M-PaDiLO view allows the dorsolateral and palmaromedial contours and lateral dorsal eminence (arrow) to be evaluated.

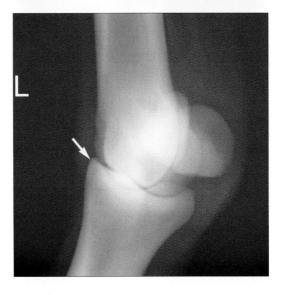

Additional information important to producing these projections involves the angulation used to produce three of these views, i.e. DP, MO, and LO. The DP view is taken with the x-ray beam angled 30° resulting in the descriptive terminology for this view being the dorso30°proximo-palmarodistal oblique (D30°Pr-PaDiO). This angulation results in the proximal sesamoid bones being located more proximally so the joint space and subchondral bone can be visualized better. This terminology actually describes how the radiograph was produced beginning with where the X-ray machine and then the cassette were positioned to produce the exposure. The starting point for positioning the machine is on midline either dorsally or palmarly (plantarly).

The angulation to produce the oblique projections is compound, i.e. there is proximal then abaxial angulation. The proximal angulation is 30 degrees and the abaxial angulation is 60 degrees. The oblique views described using this terminology are dorso30°proximo60°medial (lateral) to palmaro-distolateral (medial) oblique for the lateral (medial) oblique. An oblique view by definition silhouettes the dorsal aspect of the area being examined, i.e. medial oblique for the dorsomedial silhouette. The degree of abaxial angulation influences the area that is seen dorsally, i.e., the greater the angulation the closer to dorsal mid-line that is silhouetted (Figure 8-6).

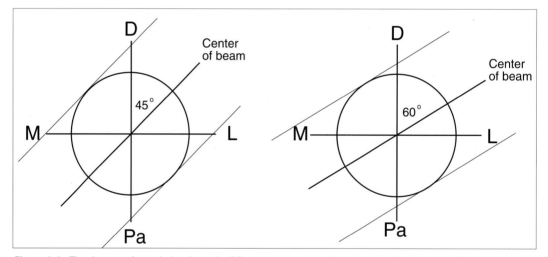

Figure 8-6. *The degree of angulation from the DP plane determines the contour silhouetted on the radiograph. The 60° angulation highlights the area closer to the dorsal midline or the dorsal eminences where more dorsal abnormal radiographic findings occur.*

The degree of abaxial angulation described above, i.e. 60 degrees, is for the routine radiographic examination of the fetlock. However, when the clinical examination results suggest an abnormality of the suspensory ligament at the proximal sesamoid bones the angulation is reduced to 45 degrees to permit better visualization of the abaxial region of the proximal sesamoid bone. The periarticular and subchondral regions of the sesamoid bone can also be evaluated more accurately with this angulation because the sesamoid bones are not superimposed. This projection is described as a D30°Pr45°M-PaDiLO for a lateral oblique (Figure 8-7).

The subject of angulation producing radiographic views is difficult for many to master. Here are three questions to check your mastery of this subject. (If you want to review the basic information on obliquity before checking your mastery of this subject, refer to Chapter 5:II-2B.)

1. What would be the descriptive terminology for the oblique radiographic projection that would allow the best visualization of the abaxial region of the medial proximal sesamoid bone?

2. Which oblique projection (medial or lateral) allows the best visualization of the lateral palmar eminence of proximal P1 for a suspected fracture?

3. Why is the 60 degree abaxial angulation preferred over the 45 degree abaxial angulation in the routine fetlock examination?

The answers to these questions are at the end of section 2 (see p.136).

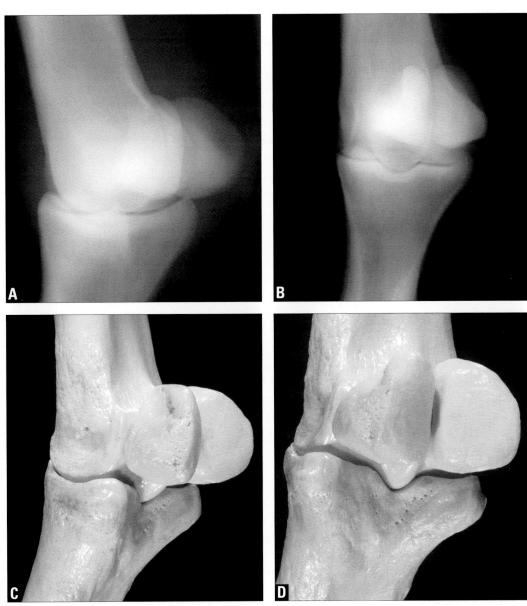

Figure 8-7. *The degree of abaxial angulation for the routine fetlock examination is 60° (**A**). The angulation is reduced to 45° when the clinical examinations suggest a suspensory ligament problem at the level of the proximal sesamoids (**B**). The advantage of the D30°Pr45°M(L)-PaDiL(M)O is better visualization of the periarticular, subchondral, and abaxial regions of the sesamoid bones because they are not superimposed (**C, D**).*

2. Views for Special Radiographic Examinations

The three special projections for the fetlock region are:

1. Palmarodistal MCIII skyline
2. Dorsodistal MCIII skyline
3. Palmaroproximal - palmarodistal sesamoid skyline

These projections are indicated based on findings from interpreting the routine five views.

Exposure factors guidelines for the three special views are 80 kVp at 0.6 mAs with a 20 inch FFD. This is a general technique that is given to serve as a reference point. Exposure factors will vary with the environmental conditions so this general technique will need modification for each practice. In addition, the clinical condition(s) suspected from interpretation of the routine examination should also be considered. When soft tissue calcification or a small fracture is suspected the technique should be reduced. A reduction of mAs (usually time) by half is recommended (e.g., 80 kVp and 10 mA at 0.06 sec [0.6 mAs] would be changed to 80kVp and 10 mA at 0.03 seconds [0.3 mAs]) and this adjustment is usually associated with the dorsodistal MCIII and the palmaroproximal to palmarodistal sesamoid skyline views. An adjustment for the palmarodistal MCIII skyline view is often the opposite, i.e., the mAs is doubled. In addition to doubling the exposure time, greater collimation of the exposure field is recommended to improve radiographic detail.

A. Palmarodistal MCIII Skyline

The palmarodistal MCIII skyline is the most commonly used of the special views of the fetlock. This skyline view is produced with the limb extended forward with the foot elevated 6-10 inches and placed on a wooden block. The exposure is made with an x-ray beam centered at midline on the fetlock described as an extended D0°Pr-PaDiO. The exposure is made using a technique that is double the mAs of a routine DP projection. The cassette must be held in a short handled cassette holder against the leg, i.e., following the angle of the pastern rather than perpendicular to the x-ray machine. The resulting radiograph can be identified by the location of the proximal sesamoid bones superimposed on the metacarpophalangeal joint space (Figure 8-8). This special view permits the condylar surface and subchondral bone palmar to the transverse ridge to be evaluated for changes in contour and decreased density. This special view must be included in the pre-operative evaluation of condylar fractures. The clinical outcome following surgical correction is dependent on the radiographic determination of an absence of both palmar comminution and an osteolytic lesion.

B. Dorsodistal MCIII Skyline

The dorsal surface and subchondral bone of the condyles and sagittal ridge can be more completely interpreted with a skyline view of the dorsodistal MCIII (Figure 8-9). This view is taken with the fetlock fully flexed and positioned slightly forward using an almost vertical beam directed from dorsoproximal to dorsodistal. This view is infrequently taken but is indicated for suspected destructive change of the dorsal periarticular margin and subchondral bone of distal MCIII as well as suspected incomplete condylar fractures.

C. Palmaroproximal-palmarodistal Sesamoid Skyline

The skyline views for the proximal sesamoid bones are taken to more completely evaluate the abaxial recess of the proximal sesamoid bone when a fracture is seen or suspected from the routine radiographic examination (Figure 8-10). This view also allows better evaluation of the axial borders of the sesamoid bones for osteolytic lesions associated with osteomyelitis.

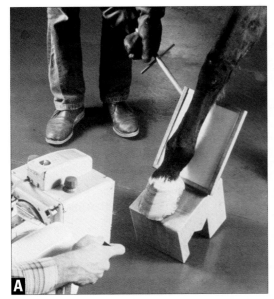
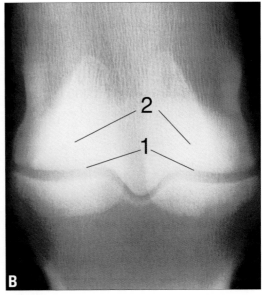

Figure 8-8. *The palmarodistal MCIII skyline is taken with the limb extended forward and the foot elevated 6-10 inches and positioned on a block using an x-ray beam described as an extended D0°Pr-PaDiO (A). The radiographic view is identified by the superimposition of the distal body of the proximal sesamoid bones over the joint space (B). The condylar surface (1) and subchondral bone of distal MCIII palmar to the transverse ridge (2) are evaluated for contour and decreased density changes.*

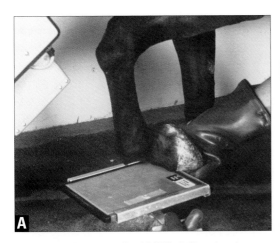
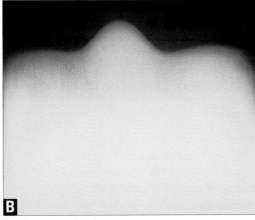

Figure 8-9. *The dorsodistal MCIII skyline view is taken of the fully flexed fetlock with a D45°Pr-DDiO x-ray beam (A). The resulting radiographic view (B) permits the dorsoproximal condylar contour and subchondral bone density to be better evaluated. This special view is infrequently taken but may be useful for evaluating suspected dorsal condylar or sagittal ridge (arrow) lesions (C).*

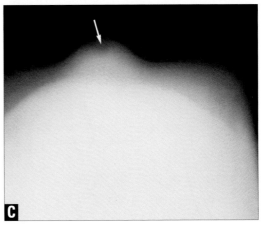
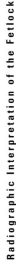

The sesamoid skyline views are produced with the limb placed under the horse (palmarly) resulting in extension of the fetlock. The foot is placed on the cassette tunnel and located more laterally and dorsally rather than centered. The exposure for the lateral proximal sesamoid bone is made from an almost vertical position described as a Pa85°Pr – PaDiO. The radiograph for evaluating the abaxial region of the medial proximal sesamoid bone is produced by an exposure described as Pa85°Pr15°L – PaDiMO.

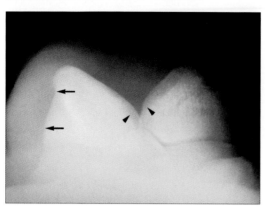

Figure 8-10. The skyline view for the proximal sesamoid bones is taken to evaluate the abaxial recess (arrows) and axial margin (arrowheads). The exposure is made with the limb placed palmarly and the foot located laterally and dorsally on the cassette tunnel. The exposures are made with a Pa85°Pr-PaDiO and Pa85°Pr15°L-PaDiMO for the lateral and medial obliques, respectively.

3. Answers to Questions about Angulation

The answers to the three questions in (A) dealing with radiographic angulation are:
1. D30° Pr 45°M - PaDiLO
2. Medial
3. This angulation permits the dorsal eminences which are located close to midline (axially) to be evaluated better. More pathologic changes occur in this location, i.e. more axially than abaxially.

II. Interpretation of the LM, Flexed-LM, and Oblique Radiographic Views of the Fetlock

There are six anatomical regions within the fetlock joint that must be evaluated radiographically to permit detection of the majority of the lesions affecting this joint in the horse. The LM projection is interpreted first for five of these regions (Figure 8-11). These five regions are: the joint capsule, the dorsodistal aspect of the third metacarpus*, the dorsoproximal first phalanx, the palmar surface and subchondral bone of distal third metacarpus, and the proximal and distal periarticular regions of the proximal sesamoid bones. The sixth anatomical region primarily evaluated using the DP projection is the subchondral bone of distal MCIII and proximal P1. The normal macroscopic appearance of these five regions to be assessed radiographically will be demonstrated.

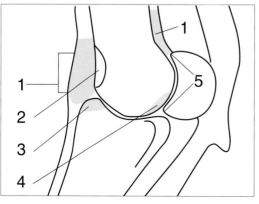

Figure 8-11. Five anatomical regions should be evaluated using the LM and f-LM views for the interpretation of the fetlock examinations. These include the joint capsule (1), dorsodistal MCIII (2), dorsoproximal P1 (3), palmarodistal MCIII (4), and the proximal sesamoid bones (5).

* The third metatarsus can be substituted for third metacarpus, but only the third metacarpus will be described in the text.

1. Joint Capsule Evaluation

The normal metacarpophalangeal joint capsule appears grossly to have a smooth, pink synovial lining and a thickness of approximately 2-3 mm. The joint capsule appears comparable in radiodensity to the other soft tissues extending several centimeters proximal and distal to the level of the joint space when analyzed on the lateromedial projection (Figure 8-12). On the flexed lateral projection, there is a uniform distribution of the soft tissues of the joint capsule dorsal to the articular surface of the third metacarpus. There is no significant increase in density as the palmar extension of the joint capsule (palmar pouches) extends proximally between the palmar surface of MCIII and the suspensory ligament just above the proximal level of the sesamoid bones on the lateromedial and flexed lateromedial projections. Consequently, the dorsal silhouette of the suspensory ligament is visualized when there is an absence of increased joint fluid.

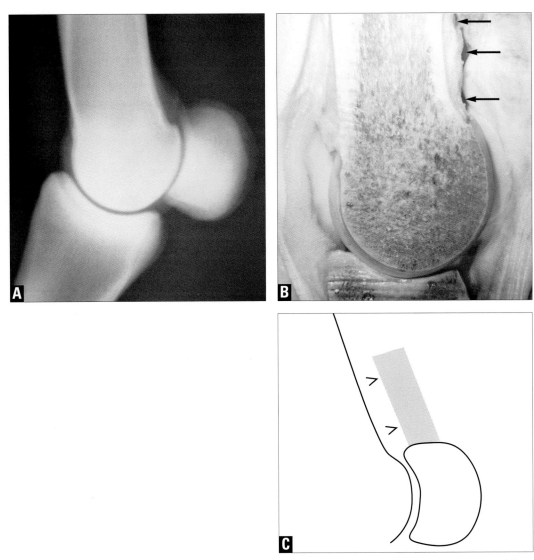

Figure 8-12. *The normal joint has uniform soft tissue density dorsally from the distal MCIII to proximal P1 (**A**). The palmar pouches (arrows) extend proximally a few centimeters beyond the proximal extent of the proximal sesamoid bones (**B**). In the joint without effusion the dorsal surface of the suspensory ligament (arrowheads) can be seen resulting in the suspensory ligament appearing as a 1-2 cm wide band of uniform density (**C**).*

Radiographic Interpretation of the Fetlock

In most fetlock joints in which pathologic changes are found, soft tissue swelling (STS) can be identified radiographically at the level of the fetlock joint space. Thickening of the joint capsule with hyperemia and/or hyperplasia of the synovium are the common pathologic findings accompanying I-STS. Bony and/or articular lesions are frequently identified. Radiodense bodies, i.e., chip fractures or osteochondromas, may be observed within the joint capsule in this location.

Intracapsular swelling can be recognized best on the lateromedial and oblique projections and appears as a localized region of increased density or "bulging" of the soft tissues dorsal to the articular surface of MCIII (Figure 8-13). On the flexed lateromedial projection, the increased soft tissue density dorsal to the condylar surface of MCIII appears fairly uniform in thickness with most secondary joint disorders. A local increase in thickness at the dorsodistal periarticular region of MCIII is seen with synovial hyperplasia of the joint capsule. Distension of the palmar pouches is identified by an increased radiodensity to the soft tissue palmar to the distal end of MCIII with the loss of the dorsal silhouette of the suspensory ligament immediately proximal to the proximal sesamoid bones. Evaluation of intracapsular distention should also be done on the oblique views, and a 60° abaxial angulation view is superior to a 45° abaxial angulation view to demonstrate intracapsular STS (Figure 8-14).

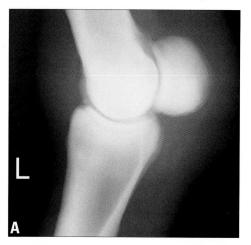 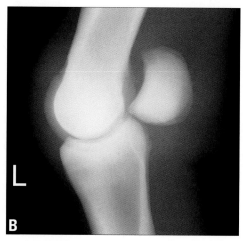

Figure 8-13. Intracapsular distention of the fetlock joint appears on the LM as a localized region of increased density or "bulging" of the soft tissues dorsal to the periarticular and articular regions of distal MCIII **(A)**. The distended palmar pouches result in a loss of the dorsal surface of the suspensory ligament and its ability to be identified on both the LM and f-LM **(B)**.

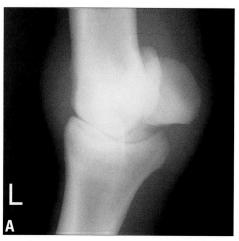 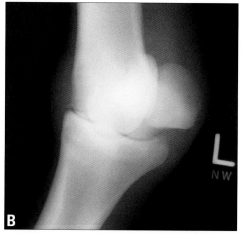

Figure 8-14. The increased density associated with intracapsular distention of the fetlock joint on the oblique views appears as a change in the surface contour and bulging proximal to the level of the joint articulation. These changes are seen better when the abaxial angulation is 60° **(A)** than when the angulation is less **(B)**.

2. Dorsodistal Aspect of the Third Metacarpus

The distal end of the metacarpus can be visualized best using the lateromedial and flexed latero-medial projections. The periarticular region of the normal distal MCIII has a midline recess from which the periarticular margin slopes slightly abaxially, before abruptly approaching a perpendicular plane approximately 3-4 cm from midline. The periarticular region of the dorsodistal MCIII forms a smooth, shallow concavity before reaching the articular surface. The dorsal articular surface of MCIII is convex dorsally with a sagittal ridge and two condylar surfaces that form smooth, arcuate silhouettes where the more dorsal (and less dense) silhouette is the sagittal ridge. The subchondral bone of the dorsal condylar surfaces has a very fine trabecular pattern and appears more dense than the subchondral bone at the junction (transverse ridge) between the dorsal and palmar surfaces.

Lesions in the dorsal periarticular region of distal MCIII are less frequently recognized on a radiographic examination than can be seen on gross pathologic examination. Radiographic findings include periarticular osteophyte formation, periarticular and subchondral radiolucent defects and localized soft tissue swelling with periosteal new bone formation extending 1-2 cm proximally from the periarticular region of the cannon bone (Figure 8-15). Flattening of the sagittal ridge can be seen associated with ulcerated regions of the articular cartilage. Linear grooves in the articular cartilage appear grossly as wear or score lines and extend in a proximal to distal direction. These lines can vary in depth from superficial irregularities to complete fissues of the cartilage; however, these lines cannot be detected radiographically. Periarticular productive and/or destructive changes commonly are accompanied by remodeling changes of proximal P1. In fact, the irregular dorsal eminence of proximal P1 impacting into the dorsodistal periarticular region of distal MCIII as a result of a marked degree of extension during exercise is considered responsible for producing most of the dorsodistal MCIII changes.

Pathologic findings at the periarticular regions of the dorsodistal metacarpus in many horses that have raced prior to death demonstrate inflammation and hemorrhage characteristic of more active joint disease. Long-standing destructive lesions of this region are often coated by granulation tissue in horses that have not been racing prior to death, but both appear radiographically to be similar with signs of bony production and/or destruction (Fig. 15E). The flap-like modification of the joint capsule overlying this periarticular region is commonly thickened with synovial hyperplasia. Fraying and adhesion to the underlying diseased bone and cartilage are infrequent findings.

3. Palmarodistal Aspect of the Third Metacarpus

A. Palmar Lesions of MCIII

The normal radiographic appearance of the palmar condylar surface is that of a smooth, convex silhouette corresponding to the subchondral bone of the condylar and the sagittal surfaces. The palmar subcondylar bone is slightly more dense and lacks the definite fine trabecular pattern of that at the dorsum of MCIII. The sagittal ridge appears less dense than the condyles and is poorly visualized within the sagittal groove of the first phalanx. Macroscopically, the normal cartilage is smooth on the palmar surface without any recesses in the areas extending into the subchondral bone and the width of the medial condyle is slightly greater than that of the lateral condyle. However, because of magnification the lateral condyle will appear slightly larger on the LM view. Radiographic findings of palmar lesions of distal MCIII are identified at a specific location and can vary in appearance from focal radiolucent change with an abnormal contour to the subchondral bone to a subchondral curvilinear lucency with a normal overlying subchondral bony contour (Figure 8-16). The former findings are seen more frequently and represent the later stage of the

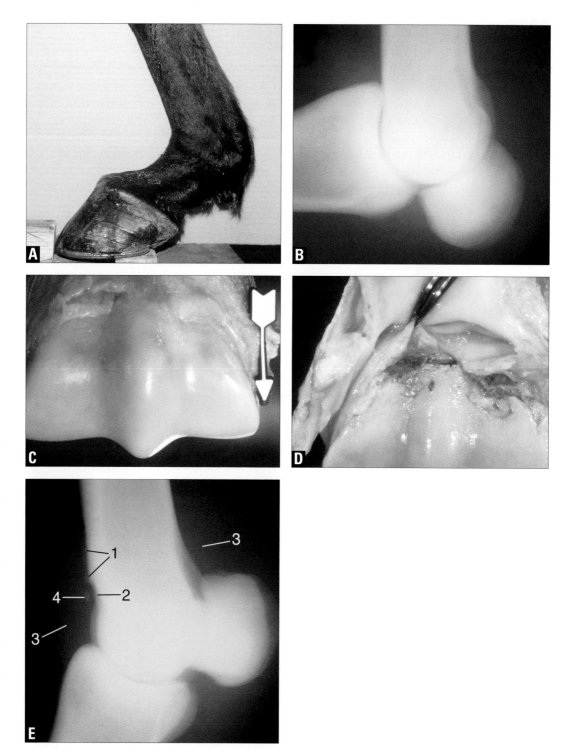

Figure 8-15. *The large range of motion of the equine fetlock during strenuous exercise results in the impaction of dorsoproximal P1 into dorsodistal MCIII **(A and B)**. The dorsodistal MCIII changes from the normal **(C)** to abnormal **(D)** as a result of impactions. Periarticular and articular remodeling of dorsodistal MCIII is identified radiographically as periarticular and periosteal productive change (1), periarticular and subchondral lucent defects (2), and intracapsular distention (3). These signs and a bony fragment (4) are demonstrated radiographically in a racing thoroughbred **(E)**. Accompanying periarticular change at dorsoproximal P1 is commonly seen (see Figure 8-23 C and D).*

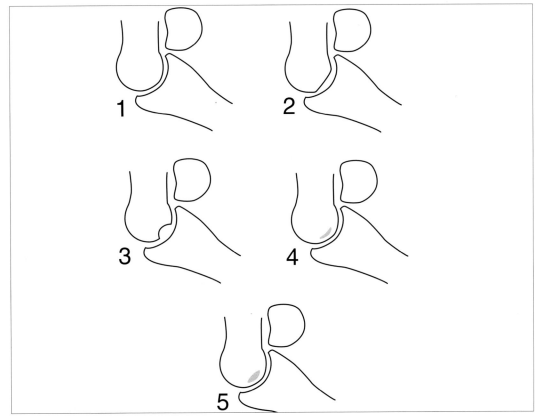

Figure 8-16. *Palmar lesions of distal MCIII are identified radiographically as abnormal contour and/or decreased density at a specific location. The contour at this anatomical location can vary in appearance from normal (1) to flattened (2) to cavitated (3). The subchondral lucency can appear curvilinear (4) or oval (5) with a normal contour to the palmar surface.*

disease process while the latter findings the early stage. Radiographic findings of the palmar surface include an abnormal contour and decreased density. The contour changes vary from flattening to cavitational defects (Figure 8-17). The cavitational change is accompanied by focal decreased density. Loss of a normal trabecular pattern in the underlying subchondral bone producing structural disorganization and decreased radiodensity accompanies large defects that penetrate the articular cartilage. Lateromedial and flexed lateromedial views are the only radiographic projections in which destructive subchondral lesions of small to moderate size, i.e., equal or less than one centimeter in diameter, can be detected. Larger subchondral lesions of 2-4 centimeters in diameter can sometimes be detected on the oblique projections. The routine dorsopalmar projection has no benefit in recognizing lesions of the palmar surface of the third metacarpus. The special radiographic skyline view of the palmarodistal MCIII is indicated for evaluation of a suspected lesion of the subchondral bone of the distal MCIII condyle.

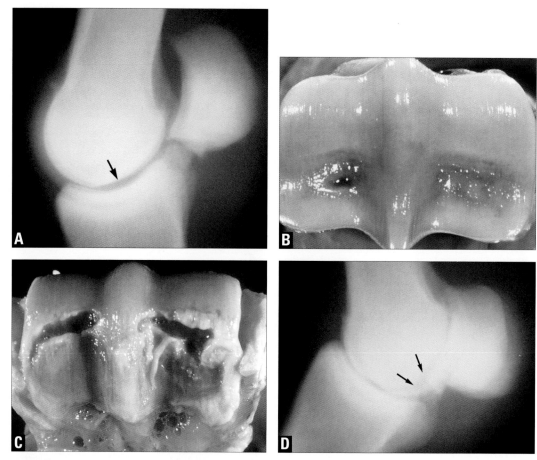

Figure 8-17. The radiographic and gross appearances to the palmar region with contour abnormalities vary from flattening *(A and B)* to cavitary *(C and D)* defects. The gross appearance of the palmar region of a normal horse permits a comparison *(E)*. The normal radiographic appearance to the palmar region of MCIII is seen in Figures 8-2 and 8-3.

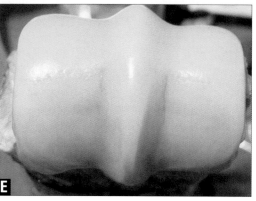

A contour change with an underlying lucent defect has been referred to as osteochondrosis. These lesions occur in mature horses and are more correctly a result of aseptic necrosis produced by direct trauma to the subchondral bones of the condyle of MCIII from impacting with the proximal sesamoid bone during severe extension of the fetlock joint. The impact produces damage to the subchondral bone and hemorrhage leading to bony resorption. Remodeling leads to resorption of the bone which can be identified on the LM radiographs as a curvilinear lucency (Figure 8-18). The overlying articular cartilage grossly appears normal and intact. Recognition of the curvilinear lucency as a significant lesion followed by complete rest for the horse can result in healing with an ability to return to racing soundness. Continued hard exercise tends to result in breakdown of the subchondral bone and cartilage leading to a severe secondary joint disease and

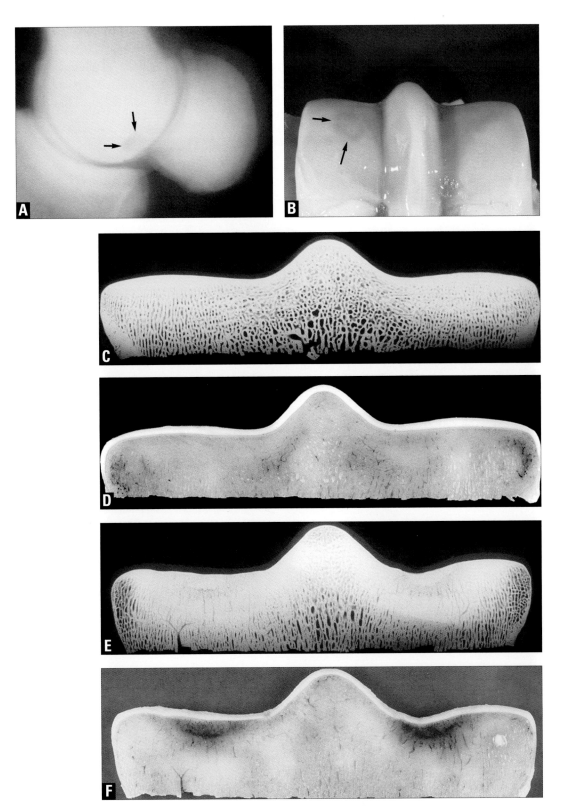

Figure 8-18. Impaction of the proximal sesamoid bone into the palmar condylar region (see Figure 8-15B) results in subchondral bony damage first seen radiographically as a curvilinear lucency resulting from subchondral bony resorption **(A)**. The overlying subchondral bone and cartilage are intact and the lesion appears grossly as a "bruise" **(B)**. Thin section bone specimens correlate the normal **(C and D)** and abnormal **(E and F)** radiographic and gross appearances.

a loss of joint function (Figure 8-19). The breakdown in the subchondral bone also produces a "kissing" lesion seen as a productive change in the basilar region of the proximal sesamoid bone in contact with the metacarpal lesion. The lesion involves the medial condyle of MCIII more commonly, but a lesion in the lateral or both condyles can be seen. Identification of a palmar subchondral lesion or a suspected lesion is an indication for the palmarodistal MCIII skyline views of **both** fetlocks.

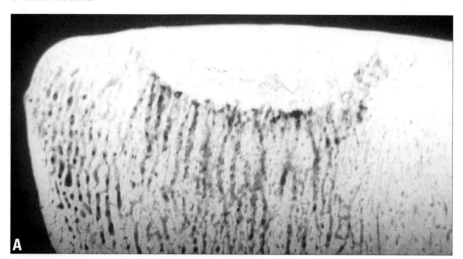

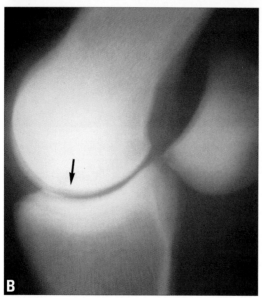

Figure 8-19. *The curvilinear lucency seen radiographically results from the summation of the bony resorptive changes within the subchondral bone (A). Breakdown of the subchondral bone at the joint surface leads to fragmentation resulting in a loss of normal subchondral contour and a related lucent defect. Healing of the curvilinear lucency without subchondral fragmentation can be identified radiographically as a palmar flattening (arrow) due to partial resorption at the site (B).*

B. Supracondylar Lysis

Remodeling at the palmar periarticular region of distal MCIII is primarily identified as a loss of bone and is described as "supracondylar lysis." The normal palmar periarticular region tapers into the palmar cortex of distal MCIII (Figure 8-20). The area of the palmar pouches is the most vascular region of the fetlock joint capsule and most of the joint fluid is produced in this region. When secondary joint disease occurs in the fetlock a marked increased vascularity occurs in this region producing bone loss secondary to the hyperemia. Supracondylar lysis is identified by the development of a shelf-like appearance to the periarticular area which extends proximally resulting in the palmar cortex of the distal MCIII changing in contour from a vertical to concave surface. The radiographic appearance of the periarticular shelf and cortical contour change tends be more severe on one side of midline than the other.

Osteophytes at the palmar periarticular aspect of the third metacarpus are smaller and less frequently detected radiographically than those at the dorsal periarticular aspect of this bone and first phalanx. Grossly, osteophytes are small in size and occur on either side of the sagittal ridge near the midline where the periarticular region of the palmar surface of MCIII is recessed.

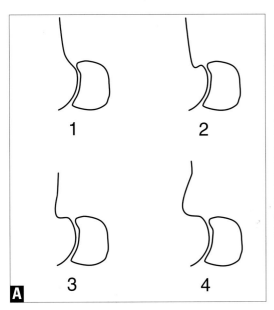

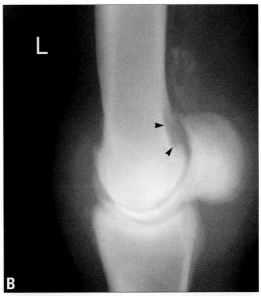

Figure 8-20. Supracondylar lysis refers to remodeling changes at the periarticular and adjacent cortical areas of palmarodistal MCIII and it is illustrated schematically *(A)*. Bone resorption in this area results in the normal (1) tapering periarticular contour appearing as a small shelf (2) which becomes larger as the degree of severity increases (3). The distal MCIII cortex also becomes concave rather than straight (4). An example of severe secondary joint disease with supracondylar lysis (arrowheads) is demonstrated radiographically *(B)* and grossly *(C)*.

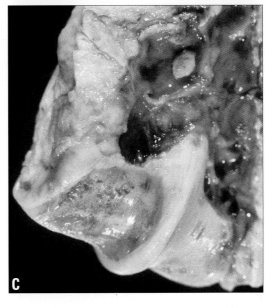

4. Proximal Sesamoid Bones

The articular surface of the proximal sesamoid bone appears radiographically as a smooth, concave surface with rounded periarticular borders proximally and distally. Radiographic signs of joint disease (excluding fractures) are confined to periarticular osteophytes (Figure 8-21). On gross examination the periarticular margins are irregular, the articular cartilage is roughened with linear grooves, and prominent synovium and pannus are occasionally visible adjacent to the osteophytes. Large osteophytes at the basal part of the sesamoid bones are located near midline, and these osteophytes became smaller as the distal margin sloped upward in the abaxial direction. The axial border of the proximal sesamoid bone(s) should have a sharp, straight surface and is best evaluated on the DP radiograph. Osteolytic lesions of the axial border of the proximal sesamoid bone are compatible with osteomyelitis.

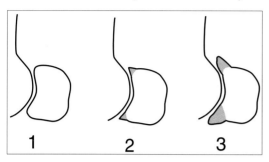

Figure 8-21. *Periarticular remodeling of the proximal sesamoid bones is a radiographic sign associated with secondary joint disease and can be evaluated best on the f-LM and D30°Pr45°M(L)-PaDiL(M)O views. The smooth apical and basilar periarticular regions of the normal (1) appear as small productive changes (2) then increase in size (3) (see Figure 8-22 for the radiographic (A) and gross (B) appearances of the basilar periarticular margins of normal sesamoid bones).*

5. First Phalanx

The radiographic appearance of the proximal end of the normal first phalanx is demonstrated on the lateromedial and flexed lateromedial projections. The periarticular region has a smooth, dorsally convex surface with distinct trabeculation in the underlying bone (Figure 8-22). The subchondral compact bone of the proximal end of the first phalanx is thickest in the center of the glenoid cavities, tapering to 1 mm thickness dorsally and palmarly. Near midline the border of the proximal first phalanx protrudes dorsally and the palmar border is recessed near the midline. The recessed palmar surface near the midline appears as a dense white line or third surface with the palmaromedial and palmarolateral aspects of the first phalanx projecting more palmarly and appearing less dense.

Oblique radiographic projections taken with 60° angulation medially or laterally to dorsopalmar midline silhouette the dorsal eminence on either side of the sagittal groove of the first phalanx.

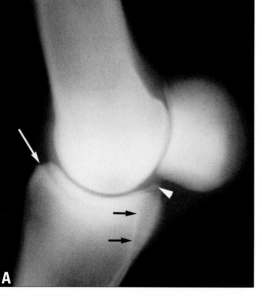
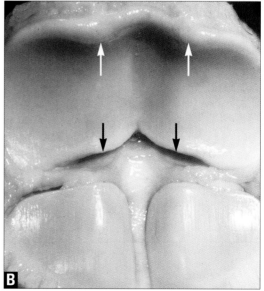

Figure 8-22. *The dorsoproximal P1 where the articular and periosteal regions meet (white arrow) should appear radiographically as a smooth dorsally convex surface with a distinct trabecular pattern distal to a thin subchondral bony stripe (A). Near midline the dorsal eminences of P1 (white arrows) protrude proximally and the palmar surface (black arrows) is recessed which can be correlated to the gross anatomy on a specimen (B). A periarticular productive lesion is seen at a palmar eminence (arrowhead).*

The joint surface continues caudally from this eminence as a thin shelf of gradually thickening compact subchondral bone. Fine trabeculation is seen under the dense compact bone. The glenoid cavity of the side of the first phalanx opposite the silhouetted dorsal eminence is visualized as a depression which terminates at the prominence on the palmar aspect of the periarticular region of the first phalanx.

The normal articular cartilage of the first phalanx is smooth with a broad periarticular region that covers the convex margin of the dorsum of the first phalanx. The joint capsule attaches close to the articular margin over the dorsal aspect of the first phalanx. The periarticular margin of the palmar first phalanx is thin with the joint capsule attached very close to the abaxial margin of the joint space.

Fractures of the eminences of the dorsum of P1 are common and usually identified on the LM (Figure 8-23). Careful evaluation of both oblique views must be done to determine if one or both dorsal eminences are fractured. The D30°Pr-PaDiO view is also evaluated to make these determinations. Secondary joint disease in the fetlock is identified by radiographic signs of periarticular osteophytes, density change in the subchondral bone and subchondral radiolucent bone cysts.

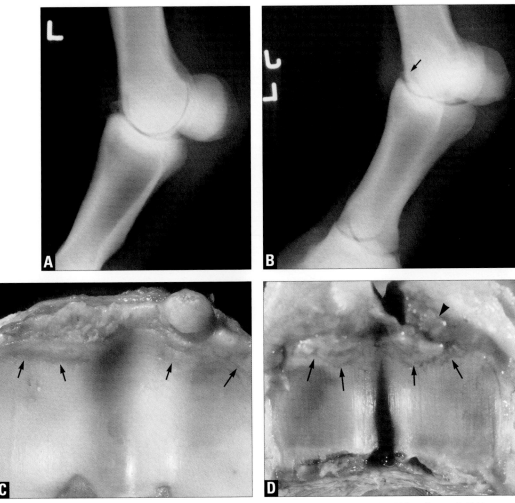

Figure 8-23. *A fracture of the dorsal eminence of P1 can usually be identified on the LM radiograph **(A)** but oblique views **(B)** are necessary to establish which eminence is fractured or if both are fractured. The D30°Pr-PaDiO often provides information about which eminence is fractured. A chronic fracture adhered to the lateral eminence **(C)** and another embedded (arrowhead) in joint capsule dorsal to the medial eminence **(D)** are demonstrated with specimens from horses that had racing careers.*

Periarticular osteophytes are most visible on oblique radiographic projections and vary from thin, sharply angled periarticular regions to prominent, dorsal protuberances of bone (Figure 8-24). Increased density (sclerosis) of the underlying bone of the dorsal first phalanx results in a loss of normal trabeculation. The trabecular pattern will be completely lost when the articular cartilage is severely damaged, and the density will be only moderately increased with less extensive cartilage damage. Subchondral radiolucent defects in P1 are usually seen in the central glenoid regions beneath areas of complete articular cartilage destruction but the incidence of such lesions is infrequent. Unilateral or bilateral symmetrical narrowing of the joint space commonly accompanies moderate to severe radiographic changes of periarticular remodeling of the first phalanx, but narrowing of the joint space often cannot be detected radiographically in the early stages of joint disease. Periarticular osteophytes tend to be seen first on proximal P1. Osteophytes at the distal periarticular region of the third metacarpus tend to accompany moderate to large osteophytes on P1. Periarticular osteophytes with subchondral sclerosis accompany changes progressing palmarly onto the articular surface (Figures 8-23C and D). Lucent cystic lesions are infrequently seen periarticularly with secondary joint disease. These lucent lesions are usually seen on the palmar aspect of P1 near midline.

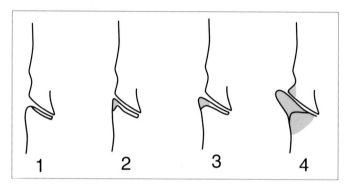

Figure 8-24. *Perarticular osteophytes of proximal P1 are associated with secondary joint disease and can best be evaluated on oblique views. The normal periarticular area (1) undergoes remodeling appearing initially as thin and sharply angled (2), and progressing to a prominent dorsal protuberance (3). Periarticular changes at the margin of MCIII are usually seen later than the P1 changes. The underlying bone at the marginal remodeling of P1 becomes denser and the trabecular pattern is lost (4). Note these remodeling changes associated with both dorsal eminences in Figure 8-23 C and D extend palmarly involving the articular surface in both specimens (arrows).*

III. Interpretation of the DP Radiographic View

The sixth anatomical area for radiographic interpretation of the fetlock joint is the subchondral bone of distal MCIII and proximal P1. The normal fetlock joint space on the DP projection appears to be of uniform width; the subchondral compact bone of proximal P1 is distinct and approximately 1-2 mm in thickness as it parallels the joint space on the D30°Pr-PaDIO view. The dorsal eminences of proximal P1 are of uniform density and highest near midline. Distal MCIII has a uniform, fine trabecular pattern. The DP is the primary view for evaluating the subchondral bone of the fetlock, and the three diagnoses to be made are condylar fractures, subchondral lucent lesions, and osteomyelitis of the axial border of the proximal sesamoid bone(s). An accurate interpretation of the subchondral and deeper bone of MCIII and P1 can be made because the proximal sesamoid bones are located proximal to the joint articulation. This results from the 30° proximal angulation used to create the DP view (D30°Pr-PaDiO).

1. Soft Tissue Evaluation

STS is an important diagnostic determination to make when beginning to evaluate the DP view of the fetlock. Intracapsular STS **cannot** be accurately determined from the DP view because the collateral ligaments are short, substantial structures that prevent distention of the joint capsule medially or laterally. This is why it was indicated earlier in this chapter that the LM and oblique projections are used to identify I-STS (II-1). However, interpretation of the DP view for E-STS is an important determinate to establish its presence and whether the STS is asymmetrical or symmetrical (Figure 8-25A). When the STS is medial or lateral, the oblique views should be evaluated to establish if the STS extends dorsomedially or dorsolaterally. It is important to remember that most clinical problems of the extremities (excluding the foot) will be directly associated with increased thickness to the adjacent soft tissues (Figure 8-25B). When the E-STS is located at a joint, a stress radiographic view provides valuable diagnostic information regarding the integrity of the supporting structures of the involved joint capsule (Figure 8-25C).

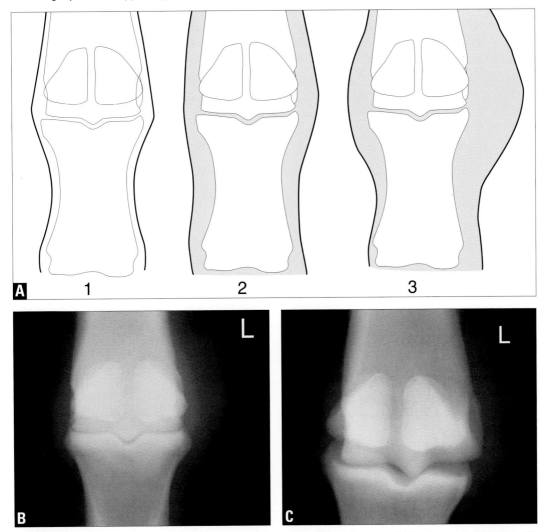

Figure 8-25. *The soft tissues of the fetlock must be evaluated to determine normal (1) or increased thickness (2, 3) on the D30°Pr-PaDiO **(A)**. Extracapsular STS (shaded) may be symmetrical (2) (see Figure 8-29 A) or asymmetrical (3). With asymmetric E-STS the clinical problem is usually directly associated with the anatomical structures underlying the STS **(B)**. A "stress" radiograph **(C)** produced by torquing the fetlock laterally with pressure applied to the mid-metacarpus and foot revealed an abnormal opening of the joint space and subluxation compatible with a ruptured lateral collateral ligament. A similar stress radiograph of the opposite fetlock is recommended for the AEP to serve as a comparison. Ultrasonography of the fetlock is recommended for further evaluation of the supporting structures of this joint.*

2. Condylar Fractures of MCIII

Condylar fractures of MCIII and MTIII seem to occur more commonly in the young racing Thoroughbred than the racing Standardbred or Quarter Horse. The four types of condylar fractures seen radiographically include incomplete, complete-nondisplaced, complete-displaced, and longitudinal (Figure 8-26). The first three fracture types involve primarily the lateral condyle with metacarpal fractures more common than metatarsal fractures (approximately 2:1). The longitudinal type fractures occur in the medial condyle of the metatarsus and extended proximally into the mid to proximal diaphysis. The incomplete and longitudinal fracture types are the most challenging to identify radiographically in the initial stage because displacement and periosteal reaction cannot be seen. The only radiographic sign seen is a linear lucency that may be very thin. The radiographic examination must permit the proximal extent of a condylar fracture to be established. This determination is most critical for longitudinal fractures of the metatarsus. Metacarpal/metatarsal radiographs supplemental to the routine fetlock examination are recommended. In addition, all condylar fractures should have special palmarodistal MCIII skyline views of **both** palmar condylar regions to determine the presence of bilateral palmar comminution or palmar subchondral bone necrosis (Figure 8-27). The axial border of the sesamoid on the side of the fracture must be evaluated carefully for a vertical sesamoid fracture. Axial sesamoid fractures tend to occur infrequently and are usually seen with a complete-displaced type of condylar fracture. The special palmaroproximal to palmarodistal sesamoid skyline view is indicated to supplement the routine fetlock for evaluation of the axial border of the sesamoid bone and palmar MCIII (Figure 8-27D).

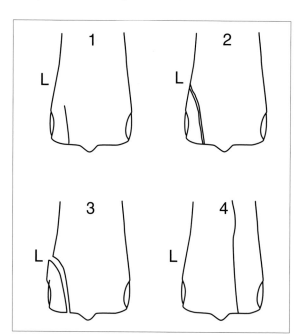

Figure 8-26. Distal MCIII and MTIII condylar fractures identified radiographically are classified as incomplete (1), complete-nondisplaced (2), complete-displaced (3), and longitudinal (4). The first three types are more commonly seen in the lateral metacarpal condyle and the longitudinal type in the medial metatarsal condyle.

3. Sagittal Groove Fractures of the First Phalanx

The clinical signs of an acute fetlock joint effusion and pain on flexion commonly indicate the need for a fetlock radiographic examination. Radiographic interpretation of the fetlock joint for fractures must include a careful evaluation of the subchondral bone of the sagittal groove for a linear lucency compatible with an incomplete fracture. In the acute stage of the incomplete sagittal groove or "screw driver" fracture, a faint linear lucency may extend only a few millimeters distally into P1 (Figure 8-28A and B). Nuclear scintigraphy is recommended for confirmation of the suspected radiographic diagnosis. If this diagnostic option is unavailable, confirmation can often

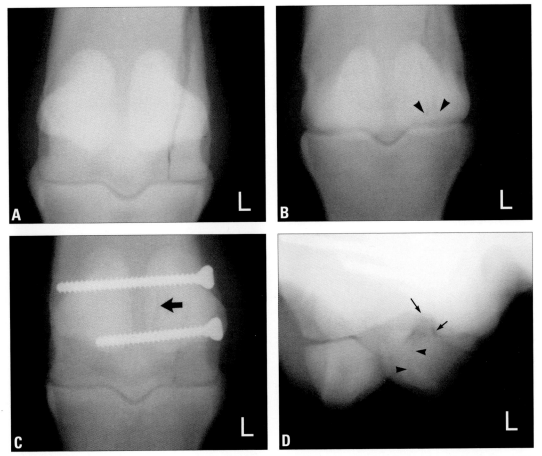

Figure 8-27. *The radiographic examination of a horse with a complete-displaced lateral condylar fracture (**A**) must include the special palmarodistal MCIII skyline view (**B**). This view is needed to determine palmar communition (arrowheads) or an osteolytic lesion. The presence of these complications as well as a vertical axial sesamoid fracture may have a major impact on the treatment and prognosis. Follow-up radiographs at 75 days post-operatively reveal an axial sesamoid fracture (**C**) and a palmaroproximal-palmarodistal sesamoid skyline view (**D**) reveals the lateral sesamoid fracture (arrowheads) and a large lucent palmar defect in MCIII (arrows).*

be made by subsequent radiographs taken in 5-7 days. Exclusion of exercise is advised during this time interval. The follow-up radiographs of an incomplete fracture should reveal remodeling change resulting in widening of the fracture line. An early periosteal response may also be identified on the dorsal surface of proximal P1.

4. Subchondral Density Changes of the Fetlock Joint

Subchondral lucent lesions of distal MCIII or proximal P1 result from developmental disorders and trauma. In addition to the linear subchondral lucent lesions resulting from a condylar or sagittal groove fracture, subchondral cystic lesions can be identified. These lesions can vary from a shallow subchondral lucency producing a contour defect to a discreet cystic lucency that does not produce a contour defect in the subchondral bone on the D30°Pr-PaDiO view (Figure 8-28). On the DP view, a cystic lucency is seen more commonly in a condyle of distal MCIII and often has a thin, dense border surrounding the lucency. The cystic lucency should be identified on the LM view where it will usually be located dorsal to the transverse ridge (junction between the dorsal and palmar contours of the condyles). This location dorsal to the transverse ridge and the ability to identify the lucency with the D30°Pr-PaDiO separates these subchondral lucent lesions from the palmar aseptic necrotic lesion presented earlier (II-3) that occurs palmar to the transverse ridge

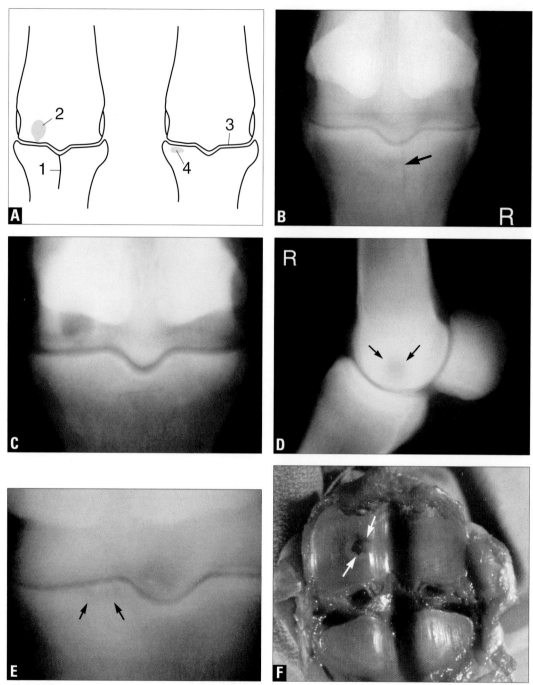

Figure 8-28. *Subchondral lucent lesions **(A)** of distal MCIII or proximal P1 can vary in appearance from linear (1) to discreet cystic (2) to shallow contour (3) to subchondral defects (4). The region of the sagittal groove of P1 must be carefully evaluated for a linear lucency (arrow) indicative of an incomplete fracture **(B)**. A bone cyst tends to be identified as a discreet subchondral lucency more commonly associated with distal MCIII and located dorsal to the transverse ridge of distal MCIII **(C and D)**. Subchondral lucent lesions in proximal P1 tend to be poorly marginated lucent defects and difficult to diagnose **(E and F)**.*

and cannot be seen on the D30°Pr-PaDiO. Subchondral cystic lucencies in proximal P1 are uncommon. When a subchondral lucency is seen in proximal P1, it tends to appear shallow with the greatest width near the subchondral bony surface.

Subchondral lesions can also appear as increased density in proximal P1. This finding is usually a sign of secondary joint disease and is seen medially and laterally on the DP view. Periarticular osteophytes and subchondral sclerosis should be expected at the dorsum of P1 with I-STS seen on the LM and oblique views. The normal thickness of the subchondral compact bone of proximal P1 changes from 1 to 2 mm in thickness and appearing symmetrical both medially and laterally to greater than 2 mm and appearing asymmetrical. A focal density can be seen in the proximal part of P1 near midline (Figure 8-29). This density must be differentiated from an enthesophyte at the insertion of the lateral digital extensor tendon at dorsoproximal P1 (see Figure 8-35). This density often is a result of an artifact created by the ergot.

Although not seen on the DP view, an additional density change that appears as a subchondral lucency is usually seen with the flexed-LM view of the hind fetlock (Figure 8-29B). This intraarticular lucency is a gas artifact associated with maximum fetlock flexion. Nitrogen is drawn into the joint space as a result of the vacuum effect created by maximum flexion. A follow-up f-LM view in five minutes with a mild to moderate degree of flexion will demonstrate the loss of the density artifact as the gas is quickly resorbed.

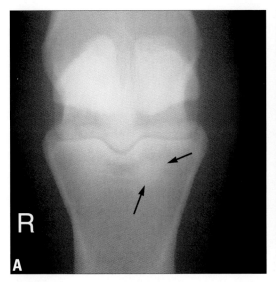

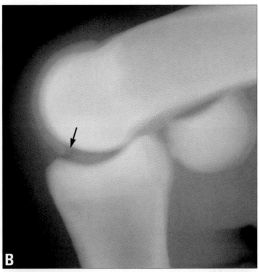

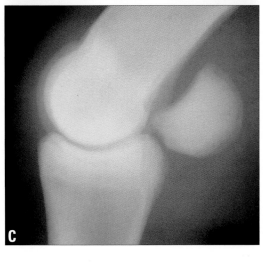

Figure 8-29. An artifact created by the increased density of the ergot *(A)* can be seen radiographically as a focal density near midline in proximal P1 (arrows). An examination of the LM and oblique views permits the determination that this density is not associated with P1. Furthermore, its midline or slightly medial location permits differential from an enthesophyte at the insertion of the lateral digital extensor tendon (see Figure 8-35,T2). Note there is evidence of symmetrical extracapsular STS. Another density artifact that may be seen occurs in the hind fetlock joint that is maximally flexed *(B)*. An intraarticular lucency (arrow) is created by gas (nitrogen) drawn into the joint space during maximum flexion. A mild to moderate degree of flexion of the same fetlock taken five minutes later reveals an absence (resorption) of the gas *(C)*.

5. Lucent Lesions of the Axial Border of the Proximal Sesamoid Bones

An uncommon clinical condition in the adult horse can be identified radiographically as a lucent process on the DP view at the axial border of the proximal sesamoid bones. A progressive fetlock lameness of weeks to months in duration with either fetlock joint or digital flexor tendon sheath effusion may be the presenting clinical signs. The location of the effusion is related to the dorsal to palmar position of the axial lesion(s) (see figure 8-30D and E). In the chronic stages the degree of severity of the lameness is often 4 out of 5 with front fetlock joint involvement twice as common as hind fetlock involvement. The radiographic changes tend to be exclusively destructive with marked irregularity of the axial border located in either the apical or mid-body region (Figure 8-30). The lucency tends to be seen in both sesamoid bones in the chronic stages, but the lesion size is often greater in one bone than the other. The etiology of the osteomyelitis and desmitis of the inter-sesamoidean ligament is essentially unknown, but vascular compromise of the inter-sesamoidean ligament with degeneration may be a predisposing factor. Medical therapy alone has been unsuccessful resulting in a poor prognosis since a successful surgical treatment has not been established.

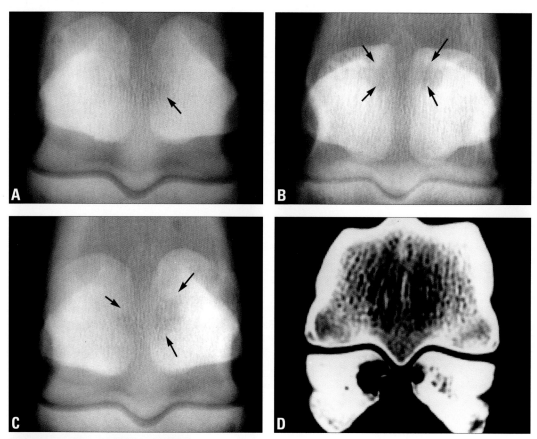

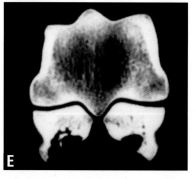

Figure 8-30. Osteomyelitis of the axial border of the proximal sesamoid bones is an uncommon but important radiographic diagnosis. A destructive bony change (arrows) is the primary bony finding with the lesion location occurring more commonly in the mid-body *(A)* but may be seen in the apical *(B)* or basilar regions. The lesion in *(A)* becomes more extensive with chronicity extending into the body of the sesamoid bone *(C)* and into the adjacent sesamoid bone. The axial lesion may extend into the fetlock joint *(D)* or flexor tendon sheath *(E)* depending on the dorsal to palmar location of the lesions.

IV. Interpretation of the Proximal Sesamoid Bones using the D30°Pr45°L(M)-PaDiM(L)O

This projection was introduced at the beginning of the chapter for evaluating clinical problems compatible with an abnormality of the attachment of the suspensory ligament at the proximal sesamoid bones. This projection also allows identification of periarticular fractures at the basilar and apical regions of a sesamoid bone.

The abaxial recess of the proximal sesamoid bone is the area where the major part of the branch of the suspensory ligament inserts. There is a fine bony trabecular pattern to this area where two or three small linear lucencies are normally seen. These lucencies are vascular canals and each should appear as a thin linear lucency that does <u>not</u> extend to the abaxial margin and have walls that are parallel bony surfaces (Figure 8-31). Linear lucencies that extend to the abaxial margin are compatible with incomplete fractures. Careful clinical examination and nuclear scintigraphy are recommended to further evaluate a suspected fracture. If confirmation of a fracture cannot be achieved, it is strongly recommended the horse be held out of competition for 7-14 days and re-examined radiographically. Failure to act decisively when a linear lucency to the abaxial margin is seen can result in a catastrophic injury! The dense oblique bony surface extending from the proximoaxial to distoabaxial direction represents the depth of the abaxial recess and should appear as a straight surface. Remodeling change at the fibro-osseous junction of the branch of the suspensory ligament results in a loss of this straight surface in the chronic stages of an injury to this area.

Trauma to the branch of the suspensory ligament at its insertion into the abaxial recess produces radiographic signs compatible with a diagnosis of either sesamoiditis or an avulsion fracture.

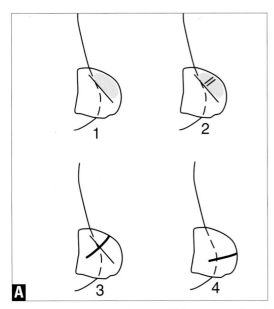 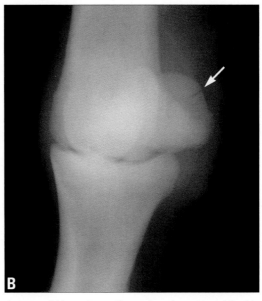

Figure 8-31. The abaxial recess *(A)* in the normal proximal sesamoid bone has a fine trabecular pattern (1) with up to three vascular canals that are straight-walled and do not extend to the abaxial margin of the sesamoid bone (2). Linear lucencies that extend to the abaxial margin are compatible with incomplete fractures (3, 4). A radiographic example of an incomplete fracture demonstrates this point *(B)*.

1. Sesamoiditis

A. In the acute phase, radiographic signs of bony change are not seen. Extracapsular soft tissue swelling can be identified palmar to the sesamoid bone. Diagnostic ultrasound is indicated to image the area of STS.

B. As the injury becomes more chronic, bony changes are identified as areas of decreased density and enlargement of the vascular canals (Figure 8-32). These findings are associated with severe damage at the fibro-osseous interface. A lesser degree of this injury in the chronic stages will produce radiographic signs of bone production seen as an irregular surface in the abaxial recess. Bone production at the surface may be identified in addition to changes in the abaxial recess. This irregular abaxial surface tends to indicate damage to the palmar annular ligament at its insertion on the margin of the proximal sesamoid bone.

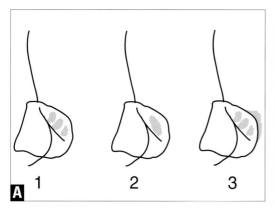 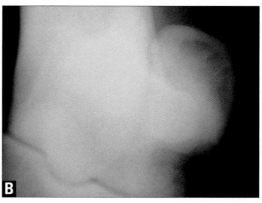

Figure 8-32. *Damage to the fibro-osseous interface at the insertion of the suspensory ligament into the abaxial recess produces cystic lucencies (1, 2) and loss of the normal trabecular pattern. These findings are indicative of chronic sesamoiditis (A). Chronic bony production at the abaxial margin (3) is also compatible with damage to the attachment of the palmar annular ligament (B).*

2. Fractures

Small fractures can be identified in the abaxial recess on the D30°Pr45°M(L)-PaDiL(M)O as distinct osseous bodies and contour change. A common site for a comminuted avulsion fracture is at the attachment of the apical branch of the suspensory ligament. Commonly this area is best visualized on the abaxial surface of the proximal sesamoid bone **opposite** the proximal sesamoid bone seen in silhouette (Figure 8-33). Enthesophyte formation is often seen at the insertion of the apical branch appearing as a focal area of bony protuberance. The D30°Pr45°L(M)-PaDiM(L)O also permits small periarticular fractures of the proximal sesamoid bone to be identified that cannot be seen with the routine oblique views due to overlap of the sesamoid bones with 60° abaxial angulation.

Abaxial sesamoid bone fractures are sometimes difficult to assess for involvement of the articular surface of a sesamoid bone. The Pa85°Pr-PaDiO sesamoid skyline view is indicated to make this determination (Figure 8-34), and diagnose axial sesamoid bone fractures which occur with condylar fractures (see figure 8-27D).

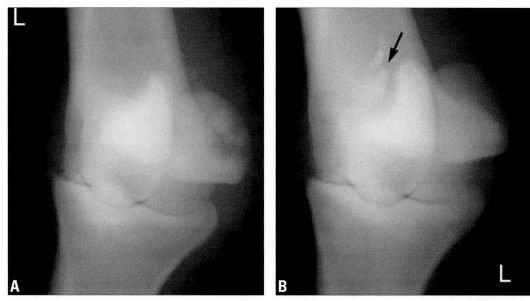

Figure 8-33. *Avulsion fractures at the abaxial recess of the proximal sesamoid bone may be difficult to evaluate for comminution and size of fragments on the oblique view highlighting the fractured sesamoid bone (A). The opposite oblique view (B) often permits additional evaluation for comminution (arrow).*

Figure 8-34. *The routine fetlock radiographic examination may be difficult to evaluate for articular involvement of an abaxial sesamoid fracture (A). The palmaro85°proximal-palmarodistal oblique sesamoid skyline view is indicated to accurately make this determination (B).*

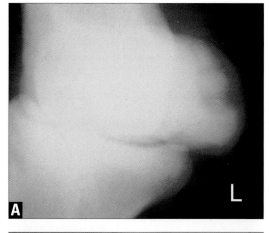

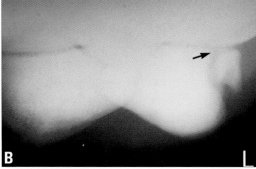

V. Interpretation of the Soft Tissue Attachments in the Fetlock and Pastern Regions

Bony changes are commonly seen at the sites of attachments of tendons, ligaments, and the fibrous parts of the joint capsule of the fetlock. The bony change seen radiographically is primarily a productive response. There is some variation in the size and precise location of the attachments of these anatomical structures, but the attachments described represent the average size and the typical location of these attachment sites. The locations on the radiographs of the attachments of these connective tissue structures are illustrated in Figures 8-35, 8-36, 8-37, 8-38, 8-39, and 8-40[1]. The key for all the figures is in Table 8-1. To avoid superimposition for different structures on opposite sides of the limb, i.e., the dorsal and palmar sides, two separate illustrations of the dorsopalmar view are utilized. Attachment sites for structures via other soft tissue structures were not identified in the illustrations. For example, the fibrous layer of the proximal interphalangeal joint capsule blends with the insertion of the common digital extensor tendon as it inserts on P2.

1. Joint Capsule and Tendinous Attachments

The joint capsule attachments of the fetlock extend over the entire width of the dorsum of MCIII and proximal P1 (Figure 8-35). The attachment on palmar MCIII is located more proximally (Figure 8-36).

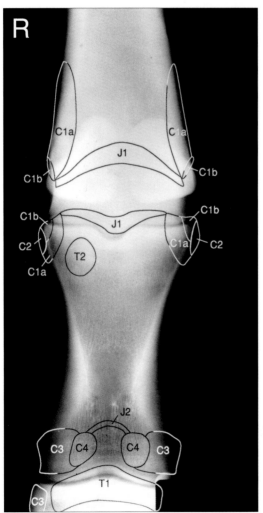

Figure 8-35. Dorsopalmar (D30°Pr-PaDiO) radiographic projection is used to illustrate the sites of attachment for those structures attaching to surfaces seen from the **dorsal** aspect of the fetlock joint and pastern regions. The radiographic blocker obscured one area of attachment of the collateral ligament of the proximal interphalangeal joint on the middle phalanx, but this structure is bilaterally symmetrical.

[1] J.C.B Weaver, et,al. *Equine Vet. J.* (1992)24(4)310-315. The author wants to thank Dr. Weaver and the *Equine Veterinary Journal* for permission to use figures and information from their article in this textbook.

*Figure 8-36. Dorsopalmar (D30°Pr-PaDiO) radiographic projection is used to illustrate the sites of attachment for those structures attaching to surfaces seen from the **palmar** aspect of the fetlock joint and pastern regions. The straight sesamoidean ligament, branches of the superficial digital flexor tendon (T3), and the palmar ligaments of the proximal interphalangeal joint (S9) blend together and attach to the middle phalanx by way of the middle scutum. The approximate area of attachment of the branches of the superficial digital flexor tendon (T3) to the middle scutum is illustrated as the hatched areas. The radiographic blocker partly obscured the area of attachment of the medial collateral ligament of the proximal interphalangeal joint on the middle phalanx, but this structure is bilaterally symmetrical. Note the attachment sites for structures attaching to the proximal sesamoid bones are not illustrated here (see Figures 8-37 and 8-38).*

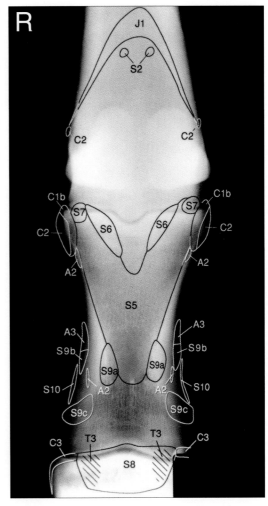

The extensor tendons that attach directly to the phalanges are the lateral digital extensor (LDE) tendon on dorsoproximal P1 laterally, and the common digital extensor (CDE) tendon on dorsoproximal P2 and P3. The flexor tendon attachments are on palmaroproximal P2 for the superficial (SDF) and the flexor surface of P3 behind the semilunar crest for the deep digital flexor (DDF- not shown). Two common misperceptions are associated with the attachments of the CDE and SDF tendons to P1. The CDE tendon does not attach directly into the bone of proximal P1, and the SDF tendon does not attach into the palmarodistal P1. The SDF branches attach to P2 by way of the middle scutum along with the straight sesamoidean and the palmar ligaments of the proximal interphalangeal joint. Note the only attachment site dorsally that is abaxial to midline and unpaired is the LDE. The SDF attachment is abaxial but paired.

2. Collateral Ligament Attachments

Each collateral ligament of the fetlock has both a superficial and deep part. The deep part attaches primarily to the fossa of MCIII and the superficial part attaches proximal to the tubercle of MCIII over a much larger area (Figure 8-37). Both insert at the surface of the mid to palmar aspect of proximal P1. Attaching more superficially in the same region of proximal P1 is the collateral ligament of the proximal sesamoid bones which originated from the basilar abaxial region of the proximal sesamoid bone. This ligament of the proximal sesamoid bone also has a smaller attachment abaxially on the palmar surface of MCIII.

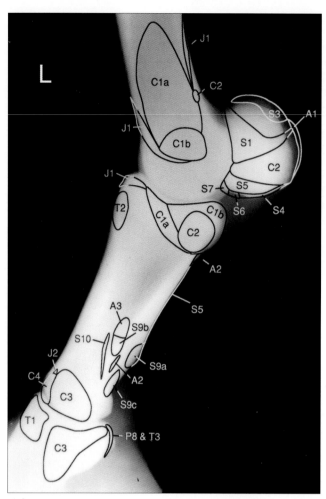

Figure 8-37. *Lateromedial (LM) radiographic projection is used to illustrate the sites of attachment for those structures attaching to surfaces seen from **either the lateral or medial aspect** of the fetlock joint and pastern regions. The attachment site for the lateral digital extensor tendon (T2) is the only structure that would not be present on the medial aspect of the fetlock.*

The attachment sites for the collateral ligaments of the proximal interphalangeal joint (PIJ) are also shown. It is important to understand the direction these ligaments have. The distal attachment on P2 is slightly more palmar because the fibers of this ligament run parallel to MCIII, not to P1 and P2.

Dorsal and axial to the proximal attachment of the collateral ligament of the PIJ is the site of attachment of the suspensory ligament of the navicular bone or the collateral sesamoidean ligament of the distal sesamoid bone.

3. Palmar Ligament Attachments

The proximal sesamoid bones are embedded in the intersesamoidean ligament forming the proximal scutum at the palmar surface. Radiographic signs of bony change are uncommonly associated with the intersesamoidean ligament.

The suspensory ligament (middle interosseous muscle) bifurcates a few centimenters proximal to the apex of the proximal sesamoid bones sending a branch to the abaxial region of each bone. The branch splits into a small, apical branch and a much larger branch which part of it inserts into the abaxial recess (Figure 8-38). The remainder of each major branch passes obliquely to the dorsum of distal P1 where it joins the CDE tendon.

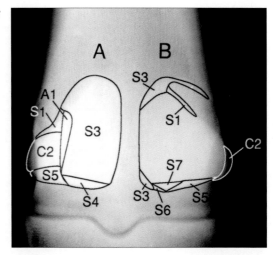

Figure 8-38. Dorsopalmar (D30°Pr-PaDiO) radiographic projection is used to illustrate the sites of attachment for those structures attaching to surfaces seen from the **palmar** (proximal sesamoid bone **A**) or **dorsal** (proximal sesamoid bone **B**) aspect of the proximal sesamoid bones.

Productive bony change is often seen at the abaxial surface and distal border of the proximal sesamoid bones at the sites of ligamentous attachments. At the distal body and border of the sesamoid bones the distal ligaments of the proximal sesamoid bones attach. These are often incorrectly referred to as the distal sesamoidean ligaments. These ligaments include the superficial (straight or "Y"), middle (oblique or "V"), deep (cruciate or "X"), and the short (brevis) ligaments. Radiographic signs of enthesophyte formation that can be interpreted to be associated with these ligaments tend to be limited to the superficial and middle and are identified best on the oblique projection (Figures 8-39 and 8-40). The middle ligament attaches distally on the palmar aspect of P1, but the superficial extends to palmaroproximal P2 and attaches at midline. Radiographic signs are most commonly associated with the attachment of the middle ligament near the mid-diaphysis of P1.

The other palmar ligamentous attachments of importance are the palmar ligaments of the proximal interphalangeal joint and the ligaments to the cartilages of the distal phalanx. The palmar ligaments of the proximal interphalangeal joint consist of three pairs: the axial, superficial abaxial, and deep abaxial ligaments. These ligaments attach with the straight sesamoidean ligament and the two branches of the superficial digital flexor at the middle scutum. The attachments of the axial and superficial abaxial palmar ligaments of the PIJ are often associated with productive bony change. Bony change at the area of attachment of the deep abaxial ligament appears as a focal lucency with a contour defect best seen on the oblique projections.

4. Annular Ligament Attachments

There are three annular ligaments at the fetlock and pastern regions, including the palmar, proximal digital, and distal digital annular ligaments. The palmar annular ligament attaches at the abaxial and palmar regions of the proximal sesamoid bones and the proximal scutum.

Productive bony change can be seen at the palmar abaxial border of the proximal sesamoid bone. When effusion of the flexor tendon sheath is present, the palmar annular ligament produces an abnormal contour to the soft tissues characterized by straight contour created by the annular ligament with bulging of the soft tissue contour proximal and distal to the annular ligament.

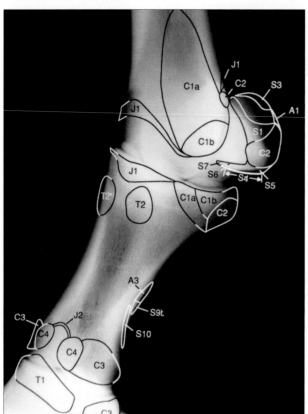

Figure 8-39. *Oblique (D30°Pr45°L-PaDiMO or D30°Pr45°M-PaDiLO) radiographic projections illustrate the sites of attachment for those structures attaching to surfaces seen from either the* **dorsomedial** *or* **dorsolateral** *aspect of the fetlock joint region. Note that the site of attachment for the lateral digital extensor tendon (T2) is depicted from both the medial oblique (D30°Pr45°L-PaDiMO) radiographic projection (T2) and the lateral oblique (D30°Pr45°M-PaDiLO) radiographic projection (T2*). Only one site of attachment for the lateral digital extensor tendon would be present in each projection. Illustrated on the proximal sesamoid bone are attachment sites for structures attaching to the palmar abaxial and distal surfaces.*

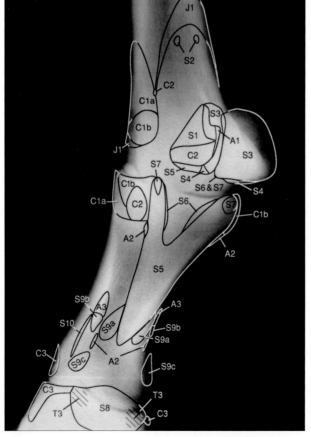

Figure 8-40. *Oblique (D30°Pr45°L-PaDiMO or D30°Pr45°M-PaDiLO) radiographic projections illustrates the sites of attachment for those structures attaching to surfaces seen from either the* **palmarolateral** *or the* **palmaromedial** *aspect of the fetlock and pastern regions.*

Table 8-1
Key for the Connective Tissue Structures
Attachment Sites Illustrated in Figures 8-35 through 8-39

Joint Capsule Attachments (J)

J1	Fetlock joint capsule
J2	Pastern joint capsule

Collateral Ligaments (C)

C1a	Superficial part of the collateral ligaments of the metacarpophalangeal joint
C1b	Deep part of the collateral ligaments of the metacarpophalangeal joint
C2	Collateral sesamoidean ligaments of the proximal sesamoid bones
C3	Collateral ligaments of the proximal interphalangeal joint
C4	Collateral sesamoidean ligaments of the distal sesamoid bone; suspensory ligaments of the navicular bone

Palmar 'Suspensory' Ligaments (S)

S1	Suspensory ligament; middle interosseous muscle
S2	Metacarpointersesamoidean ligament
S3	Intersesamoidean ligament; proximal scutum; palmar ligament of the metacarpophalangeal joint
S4	Superficial or straight sesamoidean ligament
S5	Middle or oblique sesamoidean ligaments
S6	Deep or cruciate sesamoidean ligaments
S7	Short sesamoidean ligaments
S8	Middle scutum
S9a	Axial palmar ligaments of the proximal interphalangeal joint
S9b	Superficial abaxial palmar ligaments of the proximal interphalangeal joint.
S9c	Deep abaxial palmar ligaments of the proximal interphalangeal joint
S10	Ligaments to the cartilages of the distal phalanx

Annular Ligaments (A)

A1	Palmar annular ligament
A2	Proximal digital annular ligament
A3	Distal digital annular ligament

Tendons (T)

T1	Common digital extensor tendon
T2	Lateral digital extensor tendon
T3	Superficial digital flexor tendon

NOTES

NOTES

NOTES

Chapter 9

Radiographic Interpretation of the Carpus

I. Introduction

Radiographic interpretation of the carpus requires knowledge of the routine radiographic examination, special radiographic views, radiographic anatomy, and the radiographic signs associated with the clinical conditions of the carpus. The major goals of this chapter are:

1. Present radiography of the routine and special carpal examinations.
2. Provide a correlation of radiographic and gross anatomy.
3. Discuss how soft tissue swelling is the basic key to radiographic interpretation.
4. Demonstrate variation in carpal fractures.
5. Introduce sclerosis of the third carpal bone and its clinical importance.

II. Radiography of the Carpus

1. Views of the Routine Radiographic Examination

Five radiographic projections are included in the routine carpal examination. These include the two orthogonal views, i.e., dorsopalmar and lateromedial, the flexed-lateromedial, and the two oblique views. The angulation required to produce the routine views is simple, and the x-ray beam is centered at the level of the middle carpal joint for all five views. The cassette size for the carpal examination is 8 x 10 inches and a 400 speed screen-film combination is recommended. An 8 x 10 inch cassette holder and leaded gloves are used to make the exposures and the exposure field size is collimated to the skin surfaces in order to avoid personnel exposure from the primary beam and improve radiographic quality. As a guide to proper exposure factor for the portable x-ray machine, it is recommended that 80 kVp, 10 mA, and 0.1 sec at a 24-26 inch focal-film distance be utilized for all five exposures. However, these exposure factors should be adjusted for each x-ray unit to optimize radiographic quality.

A. Dorsopalmar Carpal View

The exposure is made on midline at the level of the middle carpal joint using an x-ray beam parallel to the ground. On the LM and oblique views, the level of the middle carpal joint can be determined using the accessory carpal bone, because the middle carpal joint is just distal to the distal border of the accessory carpal bone. A method for determining the level of the middle carpal joint for the exposure of a DP view is to note the level of the distal radius and the proximal metacarpus at their widest points. Midway between these two levels on midline is the point for centering the x-ray beam to produce the DP view. This method is given because the accessory carpal bone cannot be seen when the carpus is positioned for the DP exposure. This view (Figure 9-1) allows evaluation of the medial and lateral periosteal surfaces of the distal radius, carpus, and proximal metacarpus, as well as, the medial and lateral joint margins and the subchondral bone of the antebrachiocarpal (radiocarpal), middle (intercarpal), and carpometacarpal joints.

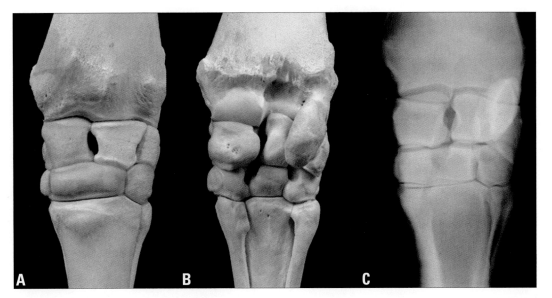

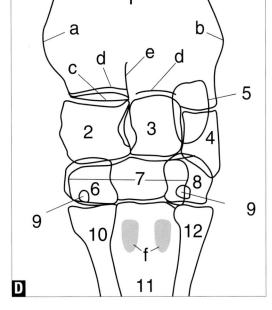

Figure 9-1. *The dorsal* **(A)** *and palmar* **(B)** *aspects of the osseous structures of a carpal specimen demonstrate most of the anatomical structures that can be identified on the DP radiograph* **(C)**. *These specimens permit differentiation of the dorsal borders of the bones from their respective palmar borders. The radiographic anatomy of the carpus seen on the DP view is demonstrated schematically* **(D)**.

(1) Radius
  a) Medial tuberosity for the collateral ligament
  b) Lateral tuberosity for the collateral ligament
  c) Medial facet
  d) Dorsal periarticular margin
  e) Palmar periarticular margin.
(2) Radial carpal bone
(3) Intermediate carpal bone
(4) Ulnar carpal bone
(5) Accessory carpal bone
(6) Second carpal bone
(7) Third carpal bone
(8) Fourth carpal bone
(9) First and fifth carpal bones – presence and appearance are variable
(10) Second metacarpus
(11) Third metacarpus – area of origin of the suspensory ligament (f)
(12) Fourth metacarpus

B. Lateromedial Carpal View

The LM is exposed on midline at the level of the middle carpal joint which is just distal to the distal border of the accessory carpal bone. Obliquity can usually be eliminated by superimposing the bulbs of the heels. The LM view allows evaluation of the dorsal and palmar aspects of the distal radius, carpus, and proximal metacarpus (Figure 9-2).

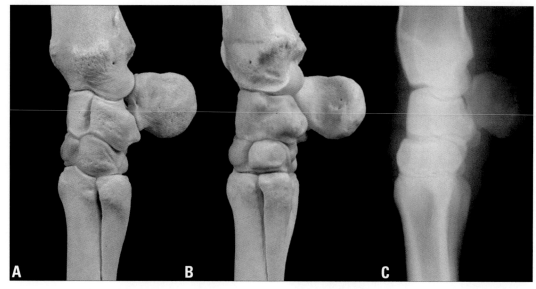

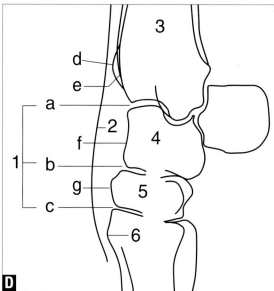

Figure 9-2. *The lateral **(A)** and medial **(B)** aspects of the osseous structures of a carpal specimen demonstrate many of the anatomical structures that can be identified on the LM radiograph **(C)**. The radiographic anatomy of the carpus seen on the LM view is demonstrated schematically **(D)**.*

 (1) The level of joint spaces: the antebrachiocarpal (a), middle carpal (b), and carpometacarpal (c) articulations
 (2) Soft tissues at the dorsum of the carpus
 (3) Distal radius: the intertendinous eminence (d), and groove for the common digital extensor tendon (e)
 (4) Proximal row of carpal bones: the dorsum of the intermediate carpal bone (f)
 (5) Distal row of carpal bones: the third carpal bone (g)
 (6) Metacarpal tuberosity

C. Flexed-Lateromedial Carpal View

This view is exposed using a horizontal beam with the carpus flexed approximately 3/4 maximum flexion. Medial or lateral displacement and over-flexion of the carpus must be avoided. A correctly positioned f-LM will have the intermediate carpal bone clearly seen proximal to the displaced radiocarpal bone (Figure 9-3). The f-LM allows evaluation of the dorsal and to a lesser degree the palmar periarticular regions of the distal radius, proximal and distal intermediate and radial carpal bones, and proximal third carpal bone. This view shows greater detail for fractures and secondary remodeling changes than is possible with the LM view. The f-LM is extremely valuable in the pre-surgical evaluation of slab fractures. The degree of reduction of a slab fracture with flexion is an important indication of surgical reduction and future athletic success. Horses with slab fractures that do not reduce with carpal flexion are less likely to return to athletic soundness despite surgical intervention.

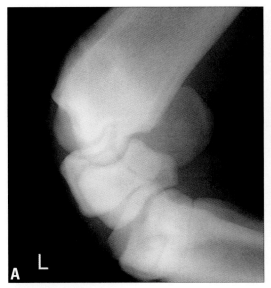

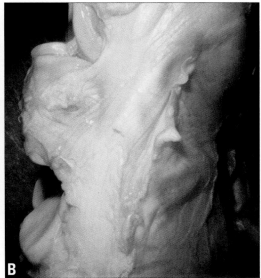

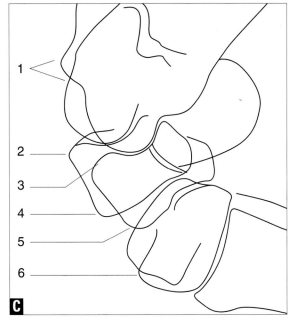

Figure 9-3. With the properly positioned flexed-lateromedial view of the carpus *(A)* there is separation of the radial and intermediate carpal bones resulting in the intermediate carpal bone being more proximal than the radial carpal bone *(B)*. The radiographic anatomy of the carpus seen on the f-LM is demonstrated schematically *(C)*. The f-LM permits the dorsal periarticular and articular regions of the distal radius (1), proximal intermediate (2) and radial carpal (3) bones, distal intermediate (4) and radial carpal (5) bones, and the proximal third carpal bone (6) to be evaluated in greater detail than with the LM.

Fractures and secondary remodeling changes are the primary findings evaluated with the f-LM.

D. The Oblique Carpal Views

The angulation for producing both oblique views is 60 degrees. For safety and consistency in positioning, the lateral oblique is taken using positioning described as a palmaro60°lateral-dorsomedial oblique (Figure 9-4). The medial oblique is described as D60°L-PaMO (Figure 9-5).

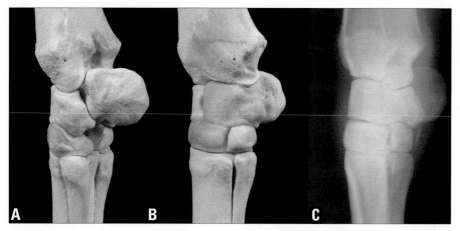

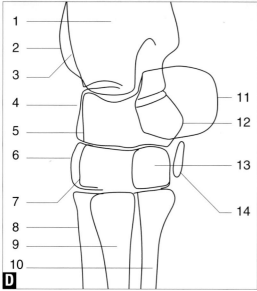

Figure 9-4. The palmarolateral **(A)** and dorsomedial **(B)** surfaces of a carpus demonstrate many of the anatomical structures that can be identified on the **Pa60°L-DMO or lateral oblique view (C)**. Important radiographic anatomy of the carpus seen on the LO view is demonstrated schematically **(D)**.

(1) Distal radius
(2) Intertendinous eminence
(3) Groove for the common digital extensor tendon
(4) Intermediate carpal bone
(5) Ulnar carpal bone
(6) Third carpal bone
(7) Fourth carpal bone
(8) MCIII
(9) MCIV
(10) MCII
(11) Accessory carpal bone
(12) Palmar border of the radial carpal bone
(13) Second carpal bone
(14) Artifact

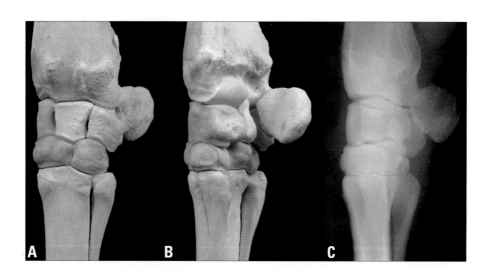

Figure 9-5. *The dorsolateral (A) and palmaromedial (B) surfaces of a carpus demonstrate many of the anatomical structures that can be identified on the D60°L-PaMO or medial oblique view (C). Important radiographic anatomy of the carpus seen on the MO view is demonstrated schematically (D).*

   (1) Craniomedial radius
   (2) Intertendinous eminence
   (3) Dorsomedial radial carpal bone
   (4) Intermediate carpal bone
   (5) Third carpal bones – note the characteristic bony prominence to the mid-portion of the dorsomedial C3.
   (6) Radial fossa of the third carpal bone
   (7) Metacarpal tuberosity for the insertion of the extensor carpi radialis tendon
   (8) Dorsomedial aspect of C2 and MCII
   (9) Caudolateral radius
   (10) Accessory carpal bone
   (11) Palmarolateral ulnar carpal bone
   (12) Palmarolateral aspect of C4 and MCIV

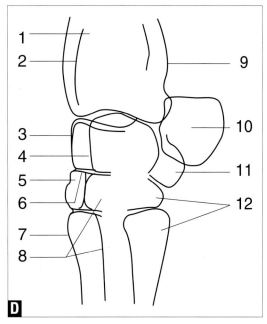

2. Special Radiographic Views of the Flexed Carpus

The inclusion of special skyline views is extremely important in radiographic evaluation of the carpus. The importance of these views is:

- **To establish a diagnosis.**
- **To more completely assess a suspected bony lesion.**
- **To provide quality control for surgical procedures.**

There are three special radiographic views of the carpus taken as dorsoproximal to dorsodistal skyline projections of the dorsum of the flexed carpus. These views highlight the distal radius (Figure 9-6), proximal row of carpal bones (Figure 9-7), and the distal row of carpal bones (Figure 9-8). The exposure factors for all three views are 80 kVp, 10 mA, and 0.04-.06 sec at 18-20 inches and the cassette is placed on the dorsal surface of MCIII which is positioned parallel to the

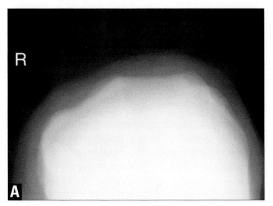

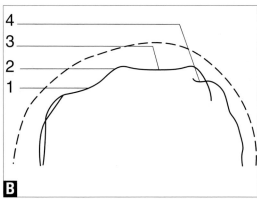

Figure 9-6. *The flexed-D65°Pr-DDiO is the special carpal radiographic projection for evaluating the dorsodistal radius (A). The radiographic changes associated with grooves for the tendons of the common digital extensor (1) and the extensor carpi radialis (3) and the intertendinous eminence (2) can optimally be interpreted (B). If the radiograph is produced with a proper exposure the tendons can be evaluated. The small obliquely running groove for the extensor carpi obliquis tendon appears as a poorly defined, shallow indentation (4). The dorsodistal radius has a totally different silhouette at the articular region. This appearance can be seen in Figure 9-7B and C.*

ground. The variables to produce the three views are the position of the radius, the location of the carpus being radiographed relative to the opposite carpus, the degree of flexion of the carpus, and the degree of angulation of the x-ray beam.

Descriptive Information for Producing the Skyline Views for the Carpus				
Anatomical Area Being Silhouetted on Radiograph	Position of the Radius Relative to Ground	Location of Carpus Being Examined Relative to the Opposite Carpus	Degree of Carpal Joint Flexion	Descriptive Terminology for the Special View
Distal Radius	Vertical	Parallel	Mild	Flexed-D65° Pr-DDiO
Proximal Row	Angled 45° cranially	Slightly dorsal	Moderate	Flexed-D45° Pr-DDiO
Distal Row	Angled 60° cranially	Dorsal and proximal	Maximum	Flexed-D30° Pr-DDiO

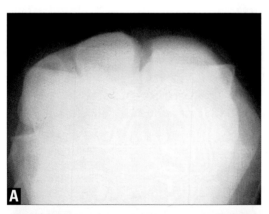

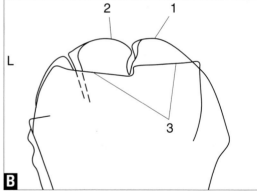

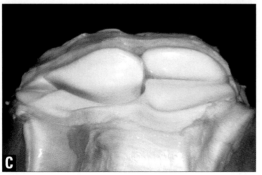

Figure 9-7. The flexed-D45°Pr-DDiO view is the special carpal projection to evaluate the dorsoproximal aspect of the proximal row of carpal bones *(A)*. Small fractures at the axial margin of the radial (1) or intermediate (2) carpal bones may only be diagnosed with this special view *(B and C)*. The articular surface of the distal radius (3) can be seen superimposed on the proximal row of carpal bones.

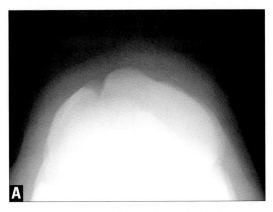

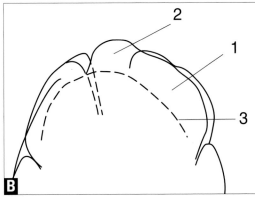

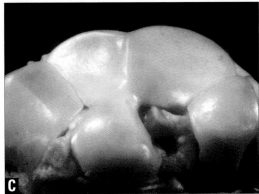

Figure 9-8. *The flexed-D30°Pr-DDiO view is the most frequently taken of the special views (**A and B**). This view permits the radial (1) and intermediate (2) fossae of C3 to be evaluated for fractures and density changes (**C**). The silhouette of the dorsum of MCIII (3) can often be identified on this view.*

Horses with I-STS of the middle carpal joint may not permit maximum carpal flexion. The skyline of the distal row can be produced in these horses by elevating the moderately flexed carpus and adjusting the x-ray beam angle to 45° to highlight the distal row of carpal bones.

A. Determining the Need for Special Views

The question concerning when one or more of these special views should be taken is answered from the clinical and survey radiographic examinations. The joint capsule of the antebrachio-carpal (radiocarpal) and middle (intercarpal) joints do not communicate. Joint capsule distention of the middle carpal joint indicates the need for a distal row skyline view while distention of the antebrachiocarpal joint capsule indicates the need for the distal radius skyline view. The proximal row skyline is taken when there is intracapsular distention of both joints, but is usually most valuable to supplement the distal radius view.

B. How to Identify at which View One is Looking

There are two radiographic keys to determine which dorsal silhouette(s) is visualized when there is overlap of the anatomical areas on the radiographic image. One can determine the bones being seen on the radiograph by identifying two anatomical features: 1) the number of dorsal intercarpal articulations present and 2) the presence of an articulation at the dorsal midline (Figure 9-9).

The distal radius is most easily recognized because there are no articulations and therefore there is none at midline. The silhouettes of the proximal and distal rows both have multiple intercarpal articulations. The proximal row has two articulations formed by the radial/intermediate and the intermediate/ulnar carpal bones. The distal row also has two articulations formed by the second/third and the third/fourth carpal bones. The proximal row is differentiated from the distal row by a midline articulation formed by the radial and intermediate carpal bones.

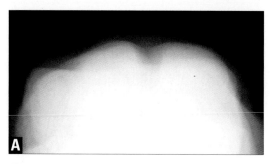

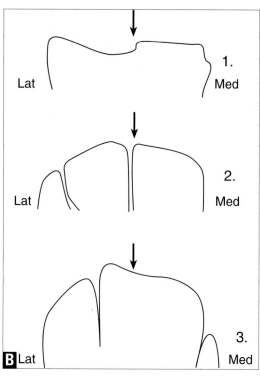

Figure 9-9. *The dorsal silhouettes of the distal radius, proximal row of carpal bones, and the distal row of carpal bones may occasionally overlap on the special dorsoproximal to dorsodistal skyline views (A). These three overlapping silhouettes can be differentiated based on the determination of the number of intercarpal articulations and the location of an articulation near midline (arrow) (B). The dorsodistal radius (1) can be identified as a single continuous surface without an articulation. The proximal and distal rows both have two articulations, but the proximal row (2) has a midline intercarpal articulation and the distal row (3) does not. The radiograph (A) represents a poorly positioned special view of the proximal row. Note the dorsodistal radius appears differently than shown in Figure 9-6 because the articular surface is seen when overlapped (see Figure 9-7 B and C).*

The skyline view of the distal row is taken most frequently because it allows the third carpal bone to be evaluated. The use of this view allows third carpal bone lesions to be identified, more completely evaluated, and it is extremely valuable for quality control following surgery. This view can be diagnostic for incomplete fractures, and it is required to diagnose sclerosis and subchondral lucent lesions of the radial fossa of C3. The presence of sclerosis is determined by a comparison between C3 and C4. C4 does not become sclerotic so a sclerotic appearing C3 and C4 is a result of underexposure (sclerosis will be discussed on p.184).

III. Interpretation of the Carpus

1. Evaluation of Soft Tissue Density
A. Lucency Dorsal to the Antebrachiocarpal Joint

On the LM radiograph, lucency is usually seen in the soft tissues dorsal to the antebrachiocarpal joint. The lucency has variation in size and shape but its location is consistent. The lucency is a result of focal fat accumulations and can appear as two lucencies (Figure 9-10). The more dorsal lucency tends to be linear in shape and is produced by fat accumulation in the extensor carpi radialis tendon sheath. The larger and more palmar lucency is triangular in shape and represents fat accumulation in the antebrachiocarpal joint capsule deep to the synovial membrane. The diagnostic importance of the lucencies is that their recognition indicates a lack of STS of the antebrachiocarpal joint, and their appearance and location can assist in the interpretation of acute extracapsular STS (E-STS) (Figure 9-11). A synovitis would be expected to produce edema and inflammation resulting in infiltration of the fat accumulations causing a radiographic loss of this lucency and producing a homogenous appearance to the soft tissue.

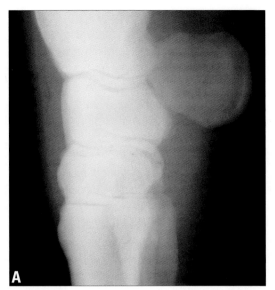

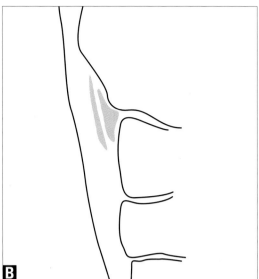

Figure 9-10. *Two lucent areas are commonly seen on the LM view dorsal to the normal antebrachiocarpal joint (A). The more dorsal lucent area is linear and it is produced by fat accumulation associated with the synovium of the extensor carpi radialis tendon sheath (B). The more palmar lucent area tends to be larger, roughly triangular in shape, and is seen more frequently. This larger lucency is produced by fat accumulation in the antebrachiocarpal joint capsule between the synovial membrane and the fibrous layer of the joint capsule demonstrated in a specimen with a reflected dorsal antebrachiocarpal joint capsule (C). A loss of lucency in this area is usually a result of subacute to chronic synovitis of the antebrachiocarpal joint.*

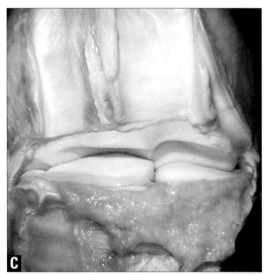

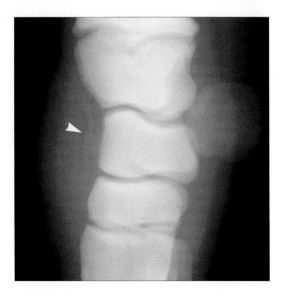
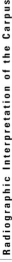

Figure 9-11. *The diagnostic importance of evaluating lucency dorsal to the antebrachiocarpal joint is demonstrated by palmar displacement of the linear lucency in this radiograph (arrowhead). There is E-STS dorsal to the extensor carpi radialis tendon sheath causing this displacement.*

B. Soft Tissue Swelling: Intra- and Extra-Capsular

An accurate interpretation of the carpal radiographic examination begins with an evaluation of the soft tissues on the LM radiographic view. This evaluation is to determine the presence of STS and then to establish if STS is intracapsular, extracapsular, or both.

1) INTRACAPSULAR STS

Intracapsular STS of the carpus (I-STS) refers to joint capsule distention of either the antebrachio-carpal (radiocarpal) or middle carpal (intercarpal) joint (Figure 9-12). Distention of the carpometacarpal joint cannot be identified radiographically because the joint space is too small and the joint capsule is tightly bound. Intracapsular distention cannot be evaluated on the DP view because the collateral ligaments do not permit the joint capsules to "buldge" medially and laterally. However, an evaluation of the DP view for STS is important for evaluating E-STS as was demonstrated in the fetlock (Chapter 8, III-1). If STS compatible with intracapsular distention is seen on the LM view, the oblique views should be evaluated to confirm the I-STS (Figure 9-13).

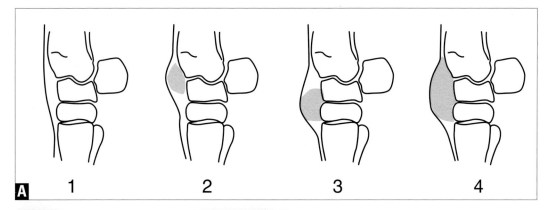

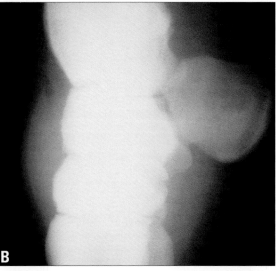

Figure 9-12. A schematic drawing of the normal soft tissue density (1) dorsal to the carpus compared to I-STS is shown **(A)**. I-STS is a result of joint capsule distention of the antebrachiocarpal (2), middle carpal (3), or both (4) joints. The joint distention is recognized radiographically by an increased soft tissue prominence dorsal to the joint space **(B)**. Note the maximum thickness of the I-STS or "dome" of the STS is at the level of the middle carpal articulation. The lucency at the level of the antebrachiocarpal joint indicates an absence of I-STS at that joint.

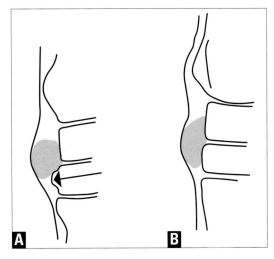

Figure 9-13. *The medial **(A)** and lateral **(B)** oblique views should be interpreted to confirm if the STS seen on the LM view is I-STS. The I-STS will appear on both oblique views as a homogenous density with a sharply marginated dorsal contour centered on the level of the joint space. Note the MO can be identified by a bony protuberance in the mid-body of dorsal C3 (arrow) versus the flat contour of C3 for the LO (see Figures 9-4C and 9-5C).*

Intracapsular distention is a very important radiographic determination because it allows the identification of the joint space with pathology most likely responsible for the clinical lameness. The radiographic examination can then be directed to more completely analyze the involved joint by taking special flexed-dorsoproximal to dorsodistal skyline views that permit more accurate radiographic assessment of the dorsum of the joint. This process has been utilized to accurately recognize bony lesions of the carpus, and it is responsible for the marked reduction in the less specific diagnosis of "carpitis." When the I-STS involves the antebrachiocarpal joint, the bony lesions are usually fractures involving the dorsodistal radius or dorsoproximal aspect of the bones of the proximal row of carpal bones. When I-STS involves the middle carpal joint, fractures of the dorsodistal regions of the proximal row or dorsoproximal aspects of the distal row of carpal bones are usually involved. Consequently, I-STS of the antebrachiocarpal joint indicates a need for special flexed-dorsoproximal to dorsodistal skyline views of both the distal radius and proximal row of carpal bones. Intracapsular STS of the middle carpal joint indicates the need for a flexed-dorsoproximal to dorsodistal special view of the distal row of carpal bones. The special view of the proximal row of carpal bones infrequently provides valuable diagnostic information in horses with middle carpal joint distention.

2) EXTRACAPSULAR STS

Extracapsular STS at the carpus is identified radiographically by: 1) increased density to the dorsum of the carpus on the LM view; 2) abaxial asymmetry to the STS on the oblique views; and 3) a greater proximal and distal extension of the STS on the LM and oblique views than seen with intracapsular STS (Figure 9-14). Distention of a tendon sheath is a common cause of E-STS at the carpus (Figure 9-15). Special flexed-dorsoproximal to dorsodistal radiographs are indicated with E-STS to determine the presence of distention of the tendon sheath (Figure 9-16). The clinical diagnoses associated with the radiographic determination of E-STS includes inflammation, traumatic swelling, or a circulatory disturbance.

3) COMBINATION I-STS AND E-STS

This combination can be identified when the degree of STS is a mild to moderate degree. Severe STS at the dorsum of the carpus may result from a combination of I-STS and E-STS. The radiographic determination of I-STS often cannot be made when there is extensive E-STS.

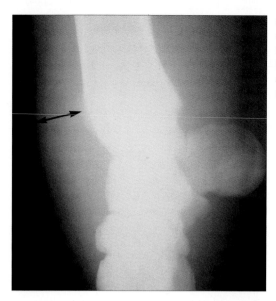

Figure 9-14. *E-STS at the carpus on the LM view is identified by the radiographic sign of increased density dorsal to the carpus, and the increased density tends to extend proximally (arrow) and/or distally. Asymmetry in the degree of dorsal STS is commonly seen on the oblique views.*

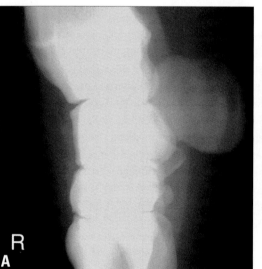

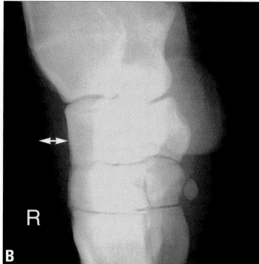

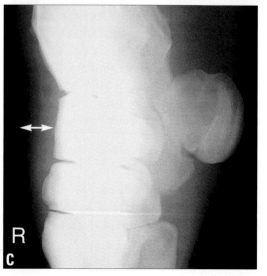

Figure 9-15. *Distension of a tendon sheath or an adventitious bursa can produce E-STS dorsal to the carpus. A mild to moderate degree of distention of the extensor carpi radialis tendon sheath is suggested by the STS on the LM (A) and that is less prominent on the LO (B) than the MO (C) view.*

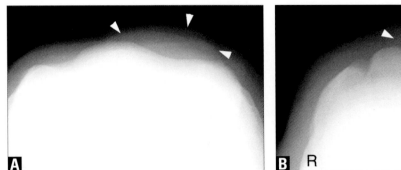
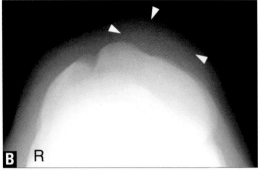

Figure 9-16. Interpretation of the flexed-dorsoproximal to dorsodistal skyline views of the distal radius **(A)** and distal row **(B)** of carpal bones confirms the STS of the horse in Figure 15 involves the extensor carpi radialis tendon sheath (arrowheads). An evaluation of the STS at the grooves of the distal radius for asymmetry often provides the best diagnostic information for determining distention of a tendon sheath.

2. Evaluation of Periarticular Radiographic Findings

The periarticular radiographic findings of the carpus include: productive bony change (osteophytes), destructive bony change, a combination of productive and destructive change, and separate radiodense bodies. These first three signs are findings associated with secondary joint disease and the dense bodies are compatible with the diagnosis of a fracture(s) (Figure 9-17). In high performance horses, fractures are commonly associated with more acute signs of lameness. With chronicity, these fractures frequently result in radiographic signs of secondary joint disease. These four findings are more commonly seen medial to midline on the dorsal aspects of the bones associated with the antebrachiocarpal and middle carpal joints.

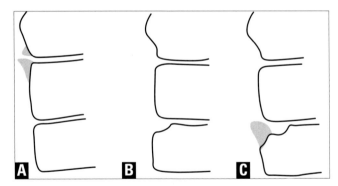

Figure 9-17. Periarticular radiographic findings are very common in the horse and are usually identified medial to midline on the dorsum of the antebrachiocarpal and middle carpal joints. These findings include productive **(A)**, destructive **(B)**, combination productive-destructive **(C)** bony change and separate dense bodies. Separate dense bodies represent fracture fragments and these are stylized in Figure 9-25 A. A radiographic example of periarticular productive change is seen at the dorsomedial aspect of the antebrachiocarpal joint in Figure 9-20.

3. Evaluation of Periosteal Productive Change

Periosteal productive change of the carpus is identified on the mid-body of the radial, intermediate, and third carpal bones. This finding is more commonly seen on the dorsum of the radial carpal bone. These enthesophytes are located at the attachment sites of the capsule of the middle carpal joint and the dorsal ligaments between either the radial and intermediate carpal bones or the third carpal and third metacarpal bones (Figure 9-18). The degree of lameness associated with periosteal productive change tends to be mild and I-STS of the middle carpal joint is commonly seen. The prognosis for performance soundness tends to be related more to the cause for the I-STS rather than the degree of periosteal productive change seen radiographically.

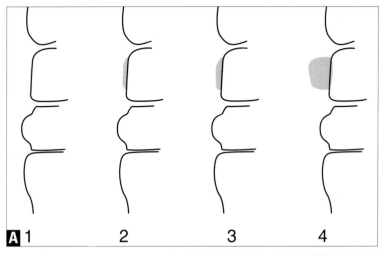

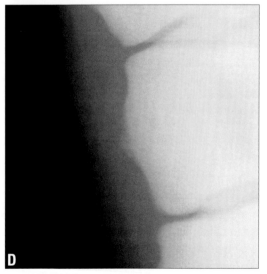

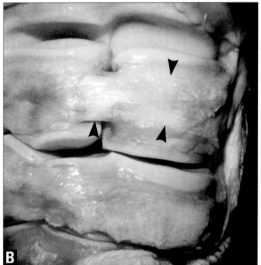

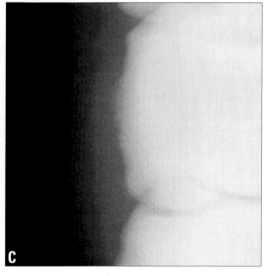

Figure 9-18. *Periosteal productive change is seen at the dorsal midbody of the radial, intermediate and third carpal bones, but it is most commonly seen on the dorsum of the radial carpal bone in association with chronic I-STS of the middle carpal joint (A). This finding (2-4) is associated with the attachments of the dorsal ligaments (arrowheads) and joint capsule (B). Radiographic examples of (2) and (3) are shown with I-STS of the middle carpal joint (C and D).*

4. Evaluation of the Subchondral Bone

The subchondral bony evaluation of the carpal bones for abnormal radiographic signs includes surface contour irregularity, subchondral sclerosis, and lucency of the third carpal bone. The contour irregularity may be seen on the routine radiographic views of the carpus, but sclerosis and subchondral lucencies commonly require a special flexed-dorsoproximal to dorsodistal view of the distal row of carpal bones (C3) to more accurately evaluate the radial fossa of C3 (Figure 9-19).

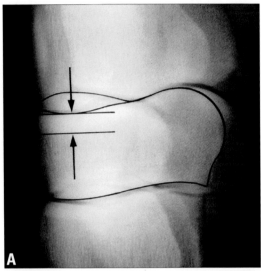
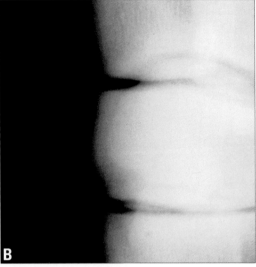

Figure 9-19. *Sclerotic change can be seen on the MO view appearing as a subchondral strip of the proximal subchondral bone of C3 that is more than 5 mm thick. However, interpretation of the body of C3 is more difficult, less reliable and sensitive than evaluation using the skyline view of the distal row of carpal bones. The mild to moderate degree of sclerosis (Figure 9-22 B) appears as a dense, thickened subchondral stripe* **(A)**. *The severe degree of sclerosis (Figures 9-22 C and D) is identified on the MO by a loss of trabecular pattern in mid-C3 and greater density (loss of trabecular pattern) when compared to the body of the radial carpal bone* **(B)**. *The superimposition of C2 makes this determination more difficult and less reliable.*

A. Contour Irregularity

Remodeling of the periarticular region secondary to chronic secondary joint disease or marginal fractures commonly results in an abnormal contour of the subchondral bone (Figure 9-20). The dorsomedial aspect of the third carpal bone is a site where this contour irregularity is commonly seen.

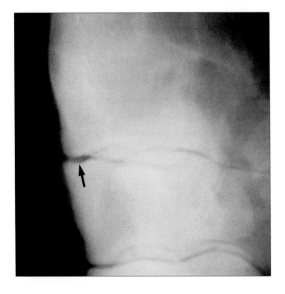

Figure 9-20. *Contour irregularity in the subchondral bony evaluation of the carpus is an important radiographic sign. This sign is secondary to chronic joint disease or periarticular fracture. Note the abnormal shape of the subchondral bone of the dorsoproximal radial carpal bone (arrow) in this antebrachiocarpal joint with periarticular remodeling.*

B. Sclerosis of the Third Carpal Bone

The radial fossa of the third carpal bone in racing breeds can appear sclerotic resulting from a loss of the trabecular pattern. Comparison radiographs of the <u>opposite</u> carpus tend to reveal if sclerosis of C3 is unilateral or a significant difference in degree of severity. This radiographic determination is made from the flexed-dorsoproximal to dorsodistal skyline view of the distal row of carpal bones. This finding must be differentiated from an artifact produced by underexposure of the skyline view (Figure 9-21). This differentiation is made by evaluating C4 for a normal trabecular pattern. Sclerosis does not occur in C4 and uncommonly occurs in the intermediate fossa of C3. Loss of the trabecular pattern in C4 indicates an artifactual "sclerosis" of the radial fossa of C3 resulting from underexposure of the skyline view.

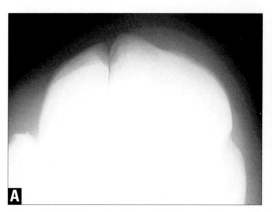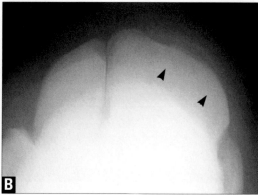

Figure 9-21. *Sclerosis of the radial fossa of C3 must be differentiated from an artifact produced from underexposure. This differentiation is made by evaluating the trabecular pattern in C4. A loss of trabecular detail in C4 indicates an underexposure (**A**) because C4 does not become sclerotic. A proper radiographic exposure (**B**) revealed a normal trabecular pattern in the radial fossa of C3 (arrowheads).*

Another problem with diagnosing sclerosis of the radial fossa of C3 occurs when there is a minor degree of radiographic underexposure or when there is productive periosteal bony change on the mid-body of dorsal C3. On the skyline view, the radial fossa appears sclerotic but there is a stripe of normal trabecular pattern seen between the "sclerotic" area and dorsal margin.

Sclerosis of the radial fossa of C3 is an exercise-related radiographic finding. In the "non-athletic" horse, a distinct trabecular pattern is seen radiographically produced by a thin proximal subchondral stripe where the bone is of uniform thickness and not highly compacted. The trabecular spaces in the middle third of the bone appear large and regular without evidence of trabecular thickening (Figure 9-22 A). Sclerosis is not seen radiographically.

The morphology of C3 with radiographic evidence of sclerosis of the radial fossa has a loss of the trabecular spaces in the middle third of the bone resulting from a bridge of highly dense bone between the proximal and distal subchondral bone of C3 (Figures 9-22 B and C). These changes are commonly seen in the racing Thoroughbred and Standardbred and are responsible for radiographic signs of sclerosis (Figure 9-22 D).

The structural changes in C3 producing the radiographic sign of sclerosis are attributed to bony response to mechanical stresses created by confirmation, fatigue, and the racing surface. The recognition of severe sclerosis in the radial fossa of the third carpal bone tends to indicate the presence of cartilage and subchondral bony lesions and should be considered a prelude to an impending C3 fracture. This consideration is based on the author's review of 15 horses with slab fractures of C3, and the determination that 13 horses had increased bone density (sclerosis) of the fractured radial fossa. The level of exercise for the horse with severe C3 sclerosis must be reduced or eliminated to allow the horse to heal and reduce the risk of a C3 fracture.

Mild, moderate, or severe degrees of C3 sclerosis can be seen without a moderate or severe degree of joint capsule distention in horses suspected to have a middle carpal joint lameness without evidence of a fracture.

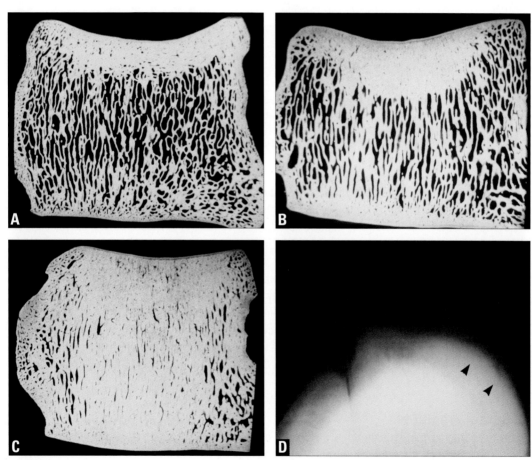

Figure 9-22. The morphologic changes in the normal trabecular pattern *(A)* of C3 resulting in radiographic signs of a mild to moderate degree *(B)*, and a severe degree *(C)* of sclerosis of the radial fossa of C3 are a consequence of thickening of the subchondral plate of bone proximally and distally, thickening of the trabeculae, and a loss of the intertrabecular spaces in the middle third of the bone. The severe degree of changes demonstrated in macroradiographs of thin sections of bone is seen as a homogenous radial fossa (arrowheads) on the radiograph *(D)*.

C. Subchondral Lucency

Focal areas of decreased density can be seen in C3 varying from poorly marginated lucencies in the dorsum of the radial fossa of the sclerotic C3 to a distinct cystic lesion. On the skyline view, focal areas of lucency producing a mottled appearance to the dorsal margin of the sclerotic radial fossa is an indication of severe bony remodeling and may be associated with, or a precurser to, a developing fracture (Figure 9-23). This finding is considered very important and it is recommended

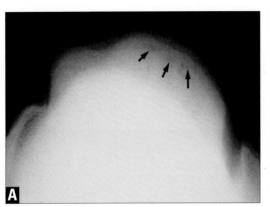 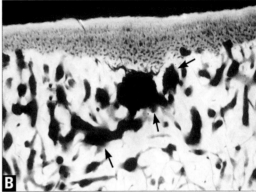

Figure 9-23. Another form of subchondral lesion can be seen as a poorly delineated lucency in the sclerotic C3. Three of this type of lucency (arrows) can be seen in the radial fossa of the sclerotic C3 (A). These lucencies are produced by remodeling changes (arrows) in the proximal subchondral bone plate (B) which can break down at the subchondral surface with the forces of exercise.

the horse be taken out of training or racing and be re-examined radiographically in three to four months before returning to training. A bone cyst tends to be difficult to identify on the routine radiographic views, but it is easily identified on the skyline view of the distal row of carpal bones (Figures 9-24 A and B).

Another cystic appearing bony finding is associated with the distal subchondral bone and palmar surface of C2 and uncommonly C4. This radiographic finding is best seen on the lateral oblique view when C2 is involved and a C1 remnant is commonly seen (Figures 9-24 C and D). This radiographic finding can vary from a small focal cystic lucency to a large lucent defect involving over half the palmar surface of C2. The size of this finding tends to be proportioned to the size of C1. This represents a developmental variation in C2 which is an incidental finding without clinical significance.

5. Carpal Fractures

Fractures of the carpus are identified by the radiographic signs of either dense bodies or lucent lines. The incidence of carpal fractures is highest in racing horses and is commonly associated with clinical signs of lameness and effusion of the associated joint. The soft tissue evaluation radiographically reveals I-STS of the associated joint.

The radiographic interpretation of carpal fractures is **based on evaluation of the dense bodies or lucent lines for three factors:**
- **Size and appearance of articular fractures**
- **Location of the fracture fragment**
- **Extent of the fracture line**

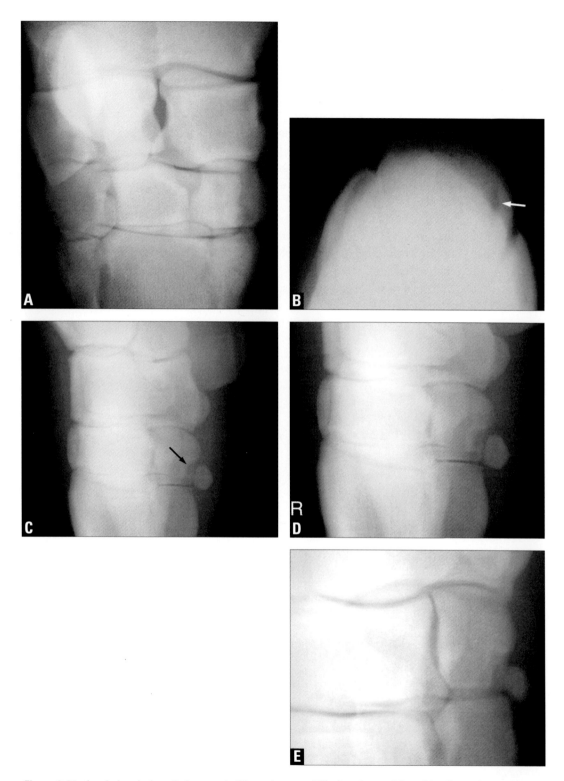

Figure 9-24. *A subchondral cystic lucency in C3 can be very difficult or impossible to identify on the routine radiographic views **(A)**. Identification of the cystic lucency in the radial fossa (arrow) on the skyline view **(B)** is easy. After identifying the location of the lesion on the skyline, it is faintly visible on the DP. A developmental disorder of C2 can appear as a lucency in the palmar region (arrow) on the LO view **(C)**. This finding is usually associated with the presence of a C1 and the size of the lucent change in C2 tends to be proportional to the size of C1 **(D and E)**.*

Radiographic Interpretation of the Carpus

A. Size and Appearance of Articular Fractures

Carpal fractures are described as chip, corner, or slab fractures (Figure 9-25). Chip fractures originate from the periarticular margin, consist of a small amount of bone, and do not extend onto the articular surface more than 1-2 mm. Chip fractures more commonly occur at the dorsum of the radial and intermediate carpal bones.

Corner fractures originate from the periarticular area but break the dorsal cortex away from the articular margin often near the attachment of the fibrous layer of the joint capsule. When compared to chip fractures, they have a larger body of bone and extend more palmarly onto the articular surface. Corner fractures are seen more commonly at the dorsum of the distal radius and proximal C3.

Slab fractures extend from one articular surface to the opposite one, originate more palmarly than chip and most corner fractures, and are commonly seen in C3. Uncommonly slab fractures are seen in the radial carpal bone.

This description based on size and appearance is subjective and has some limitations. This is apparent when one considers the differentiation of a large chip fracture from a small corner fracture. However, most carpal fractures can be accurately differentiated using these descriptive terms.

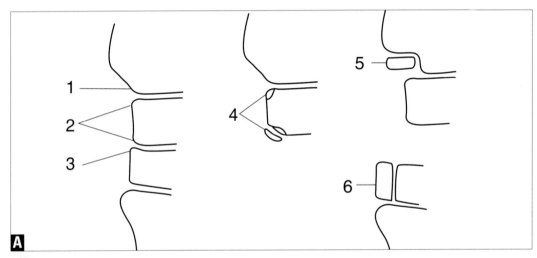

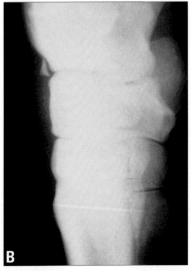

Figure 9-25. Carpal bone fractures **(A)** are commonly identified radiographically at the dorsum of the distal radius (1), proximal and distal radial and intermediate carpal bones (2) and the proximal third carpal bone (3). These fractures are described radiographically based on size and appearance as chip (4), corner (5), or slab fractures (6). However, it is important to realize that overlap exists when describing a fracture as either a large chip or a small corner **(B)**. This dense, sharply marginated osseous body from the distal radius represents the appearance of an acute fracture that could be described as either a large chip or small corner fracture.

B. Location of the Fragment

An important radiographic consideration is where the fracture fragment is located relative to its origin. The fracture fragment is described as displaced or non-displaced. This radiographic determination must be considered with size and appearance because of the implication for treatment. A non-displaced chip fracture may be treated conservatively, but a displaced slab fracture requires surgical treatment. In addition, a complete fracture should be carefully evaluated on the flexed-LM radiograph when surgical reduction is considered to determine the degree of reduction of the fragment with flexion.

C. Extent of the Fracture

A radiographic interpretation of the fracture must be done to determine if it is complete or incomplete and simple or comminuted. Determination of extent is usually associated with C3. The flexed-dorsoproximal to dorsodistal skyline view of C3 is extremely valuable to make these radiographic determinations (Figure 9-26).

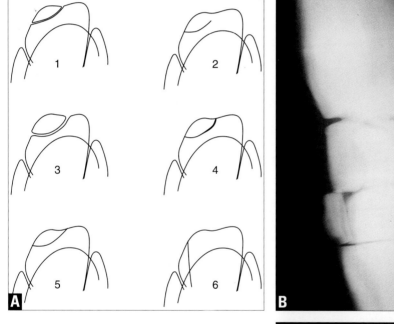

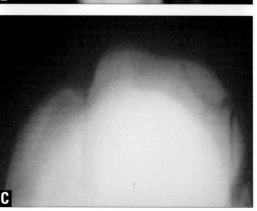

Figure 9-26. The radiographic appearance of C3 fractures on the flexed skyline view of the distal row has been stylized to demonstrate the importance of analyzing the location and extent of lucent lines and dense bodies (**A**). Radiographic differentiations should be made between a complete (1) and an incomplete (2) fracture, a displaced (3) and non-displaced (4) fracture, and an oblique (5) and a sagittal (6) fracture. The interpretation of both routine and special radiographic views is important for accuracy and completeness. A complete, displaced slab fracture of the dorsomedial C3 is easily visualized on the MO view (**B**). The skyline view of C3 permitted comminution of the fracture to be determined. The dorsal point of comminution is at the location where a screw would be placed to stabilize a simple slab fracture (**C**).

6. Palmaroproximal MCIII

Another important evaluation made from the DP and oblique views of the carpus is the diagnosis of radiographic abnormalities of the palmar region of proximal MCIII at the origin of the suspensory ligament. The attachment sites of the normal medial and lateral heads of the suspensory ligament are associated with a fine trabecular pattern in MCIII that is uniform in density from medial to lateral (Figure 9-27). Damage to the origin of the suspensory ligament can be identified as bony remodeling or as a fracture line in MCIII.

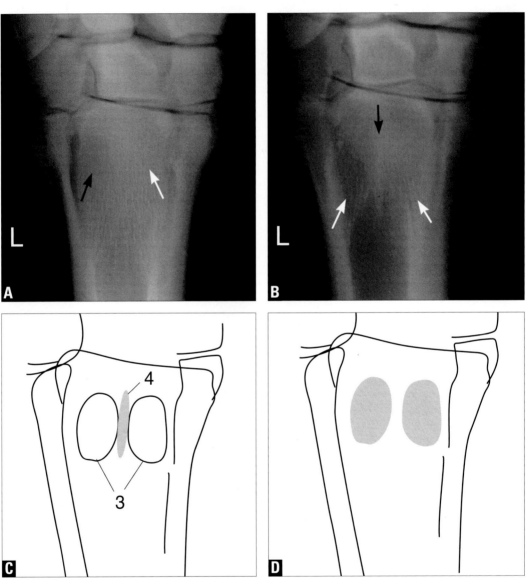

Figure 9-27. *The carpal radiographic examination permits the palmaroproximal MCIII to be evaluated for evidence of bony change at the origin of the medial (white arrowhead) and lateral (black arrowhead) heads of the suspensory ligament **(A)**. The normal trabecular pattern should be fine and uniform medially and laterally with no evidence of linear lucencies. Radiographic findings associated with bony remodeling of palmaroproximal MCIII without evidence of a fracture **(B and C)** include: increased lucency associated with resorption identified as a coarser trabecular pattern (3), and a midline linear density (4) produced by the unresorbed bone between the sites of attachment of the two heads of the suspensory ligament. As the clinical condition becomes more chronic, remodeling occurs identified as increased density and periosteal reaction **(D)**. This latter remodeling finding is usually seen on the lateral oblique view at the origin of the medial head of the suspensory ligament.*

The bony remodeling results in resorption that may involve one or both heads, a midline linear density extending proximally to distally, and/or a mild degree of periosteal reaction surrounding a lucency created by bony resorption. The area of origin of the medial head is more commonly associated with these remodeling changes. Most of these radiographic findings are best visualized on the DP view, but the periosteal reaction may be seen best on the oblique view.

Avulsion fractures at the palmaroproximal MCIII are usually identified on the DP view. These fractures appear as lucent linear findings and tend to be extensive involving attachment sites of both heads of the suspensory ligament (Figure 9-28). When the fracture is associated with a single head of the suspensory ligament, it is usually the medial one. Identification of a palmarly displaced avulsed fracture fragment is uncommon and careful interpretation of the oblique views is required (Figure 9-29). The loss of the lucent linear fracture lines associated with radiographic evidences of complete healing takes an extensive time…sometimes more than a year.

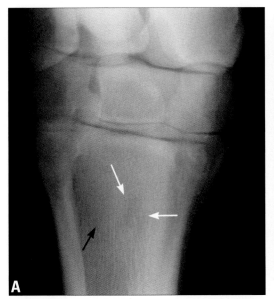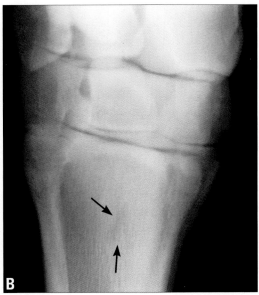

Figure 9-28. An avulsion fracture in palmaroproximal MCIII is usually identified as a linear lucency involving the area of attachment of both *(A)* or one *(B)* head of the suspensory ligament.

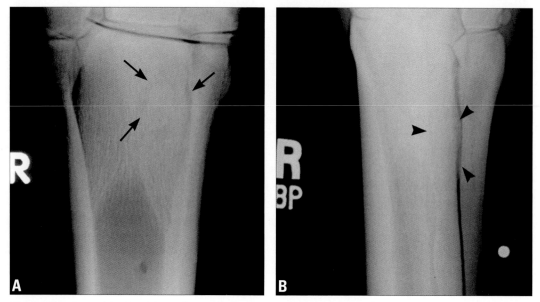

Figure 9-29. *An avulsion involving only one head of the suspensory ligament (arrows) will usually be seen medially and uncommonly will be displaced **(A)**. Lateral oblique views at different degrees of angulation may be needed to demonstrate displacement **(B)**. Ultrasonographic evaluation is also recommended.*

NOTES

NOTES

NOTES

NOTES

Chapter 10

Radiographic Interpretation of the Tarsus

I. Introduction

II. Radiography of the Tarsus
1. Views of the Routine Tarsal Examination
2. Special Radiographic Views of the Tarsus
3. Exposure Factors

III. Interpretation of the Tarsus
1. Soft Tissue Swelling (STS) Without Bony Changes
2. Secondary Joint Disease
3. Fractures
4. Infection
5. Developmental Orthopedic Disease
   A. OCD of the Intermediate Ridge of the Tibia
   B. OCD of the Ridge of the Trochlea of the Talus
   C. Absence of Normal Trabecular Pattern at the Dorsum of the Central and/or Third Tarsal Bones

I. Introduction

Tarsal diseases are a common cause of hind limb lameness in the horse. The clinical signs of tarsal disease often resemble those of stifle disease particularly the response to flexion tests. As a result both the stifle and tarsus are commonly radiographed to identify pathologic change in the horse with a hind limb lameness and during purchase evaluations. It seems prudent for purchase evaluations to radiograph these anatomical areas in both limbs.

Radiographic interpretation of the tarsus is considered difficult by most equine practitioners. There seems to be three major causes of this difficulty. These are (1) the numerous bones comprising the tarsus, (2) the variety of shapes of the tarsal bones, and (3) veterinarians tend to be less familiar with the radiographic anatomy and pathology of the tarsus than most other anatomical regions, particularly regions of the fore limb.

I am going to make some general statements in an attempt to simplify the radiographic interpretation of the tarsus. These general statements are:
- **Most radiographic findings are located at the dorsum of the tarsus.**
- **Pathologic abnormalities of the tarsus tend to be in specific anatomical areas. Soft tissue swelling (STS) is a key for assisting to localize the abnormality.**
- **There are only a few radiographic diagnoses for the tarsus.**
- **The diagnoses of abnormalities of the tarsus identified with radiology can be classified in the following way:**
  1. **Soft tissue swelling without bony change**
  2. **Secondary joint disease**
  3. **Fractures**
  4. **Infection**
  5. **Osteochondrosis and developmental disorders**
- **The radiographic findings of these five conditions will be correlated to gross pathologic findings to explain the radiographic signs and their variations.**

II. Radiography of the Tarsus

1. Views of the Routine Tarsal Examination: Four
The standard or routine radiographic examination of the equine tarsus should consist of at least four projections. These projections are:
- **Dorso0°proximal-plantarodistal oblique or dorsoplantar (DPI)**
- **Latero3°proximal-mediodistal oblique or lateromedial (LM)**
- **Dorso45°lateral-plantaromedial oblique or medial oblique (MO)**
- **Plantaro5°disto60°lateral-dorsoproximomedial oblique or lateral oblique (LO)**

A. The Dorsoplantar View
- Centering the DPI View - The foot is positioned with the toe pointing slightly laterally to assist with positioning the x-ray machine. The beam is centered at the central tarsal bone (middle of the tarsus) and directed from the dorso0°proximal to plantarodistal (Figure 10-1).

The DPI view should be taken at 0° proximally because this angulation opens the medial aspect of the intertarsal joint spaces where most signs of secondary joint disease are located. Proximal angulation of 10-15° opens in the lateral aspect of the intertarsal joint spaces with loss of the

Figure 10-1. *The foot is positioned with toe slightly lateral to produce the dorso0°proximal-plantarodistal oblique (DPI). The beam is centered on midline at the central tarsal bone.*

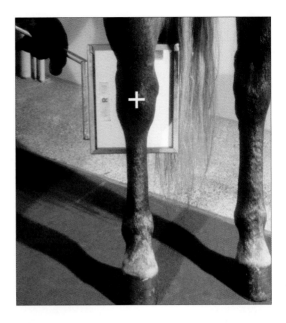

medial aspect of these joint spaces (Figure 10-2). This information is important if there is change suspected on the lateral side of midline in the tarsus. Angulation can be determined from the radiograph by the location of the head of MT IV relative to the distal intertarsal joint (DIT) space, i.e., the closer the two indicates greater proximal angulation and the further MT IV is from the DIT joint space the closer to 0° proximal angulation.

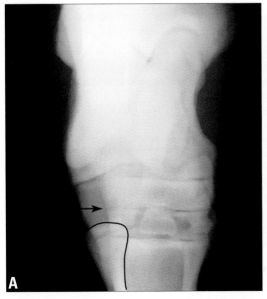
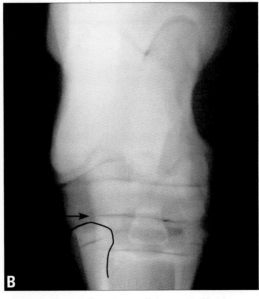

Figure 10-2. *The routine DPI view is taken without proximal angulation to allow the medial aspect of both intertarsals and the tarsometatarsal joint spaces to be interpreted because this is where most pathological changes are seen **(A)**. Proximal angulation of 10-15° highlights the lateral aspect of these joints **(B)**. Angulation can be determined by the location of the head of MT IV relative to the distal intertarsal joint space, i.e., the "higher" the head, the greater the degree of angulation.*

- Primary anatomical areas of the tarsus identified radiographically (Figure 10-3) with the DPI view are:
  - Medial and lateral surfaces and cortices of the distal tibia, tarsus, and proximal metatarsus.
  - Periarticular and subchondral regions of the four major joints of the tarsus.
  - Thickness (proximodistal height) of the central and third tarsal bones and the medial versus lateral parts of each bone (both should be comparable).
  - Location of the head of MT IV relative to the lateral aspect of the DIT space.
  - Intertarsal and TMT joint space widths on a well-positioned radiograph should be comparable.
  - Proximal tuberosity and distal tuberosity of the talus.
  - Distal region of the lateral ridge of the trochlea of the talus.
  - Plantar region of the central tarsal bone.
  - Area of origin of the suspensory ligament on plantaroproximal MT III.

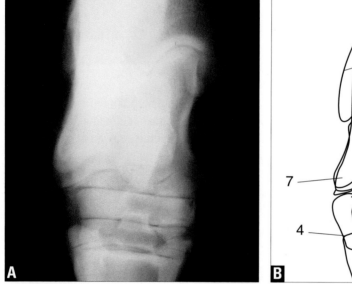 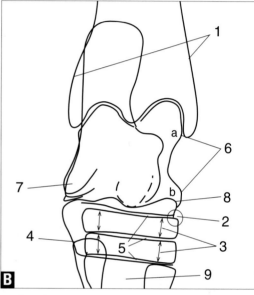

Figure 10-3. The DPI radiographic *(A)* view allows interpretation of:
  (1) The medial and lateral surfaces and cortices of the distal tibia, tarsus, and proximal metatarsus (B).
  (2) Periarticular and subchondral regions of the four major joints of the tarsus
  (3) The thickness (proximodistal height) of the central and third tarsal bones and the medial versus lateral parts of each bones (both should be comparable).
  (4) Location of the head of MT IV relative to the lateral aspect of the DIT joint space. This relationship must be correlated to joint space width.
  (5) On a well-positioned radiograph, the intertarsal and TMT joint spaces width should be comparable.
  (6) The proximal tuberosity (a) and distal tuberosity (b) of the talus.
  (7) Distal region of the lateral ridge of the trochlea of the talus.
  (8) Plantar border of the central tarsal bone.
  (9) Area of origin of the suspensory ligament on plantaroproximal MT III.

B. The Lateromedial View

Centering the LM View - The heels are superimposed to produce a true LM view where the ridges of the trochlea of the talus are superimposed. The x-ray beam is centered at the level of the central tarsal bone and there is a slight (3-5°) downward angulation of the beam resulting in the accurate descriptive name for this view being a latero3°proximal-mediodistal oblique (Figure 10-4).

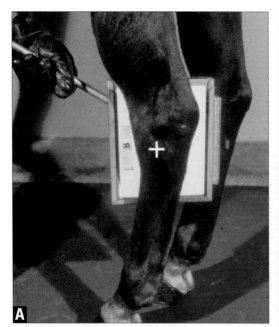

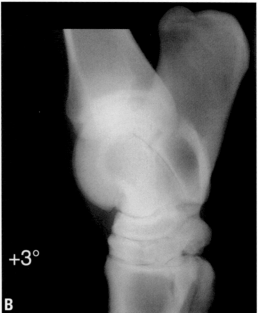

+3°

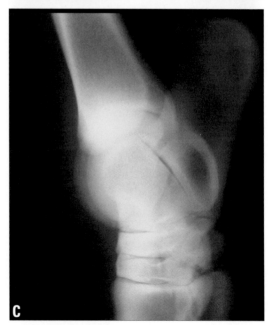

Figure 10-4. *The LM view is produced with an x-ray beam centered at the central tarsal bone and directed as a latero 3° proximal-mediodistal oblique (**A**). This angulation results in the dorsal aspect of the distal intertarsal joint space being better seen (**B and C**).*

- Primary anatomical area of the tarsus identified radiographically (Figure 10-5) with the LM view are:
  - Dorsal and plantar surfaces and cortices of the distal tibia, tarsus, and proximal metatarsus.
  - Soft tissue swelling, especially intracapsular STS of the tarsocrural joint.
  - Medial ridge of the trochlea of the talus.
  - Lateral ridge of the trochlea of the talus.
  - Dorsal region of the intermediate ridge.
  - Contour of the sustentaculum tali.
  - Periarticular and subchondral regions of the four major joints of the tarsus.
  - Dorsal surface to the central and third tarsal bones. An imaginary straight line connecting the periarticular regions of the dorsodistal talus and the dorsoproximal MT III should be envisioned. Bone dorsal to this line on the LM view represents a productive change.
  - Comparable proximodistal thickness of the central and third tarsal bones.

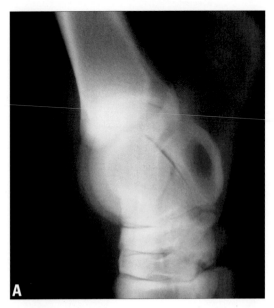

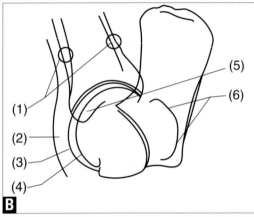

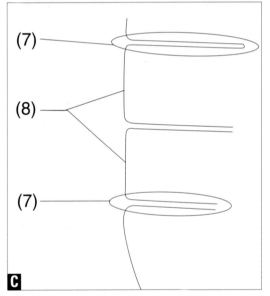

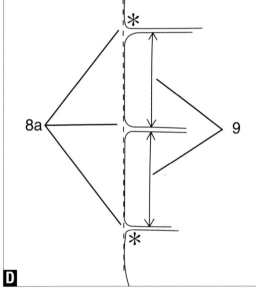

Figure 10-5. The LM radiographic view *(A)* allows interpretation of:

(1) Dorsal and plantar surfaces and cortices of the distal tibia, tarsus, and proximal metatarsus *(B)*.

(2) Soft tissue swelling, especially intracapsular STS of the tarsocrural joint.

(3) Medial ridge of the trochlea of the talus.

(4) Lateral ridge of the trochlea of the talus.

(5) Dorsal region of the intermediate ridge.

(6) Contour of the sustentaculum tali.

(7) Periarticular and subchondral regions of the four major joints of the tarsus *(C)*.

(8) Dorsal surfaces of the central and third tarsal bones. An imaginary straight line (8a) connecting the periarticular regions (asterisks) of the dorsodistal talus and the dorsoproximal MT III should be envisioned *(D)*. Bone dorsal to this line on the LM view represents a productive change. This determination is made on the LM view and not the oblique views. The third tarsal bone's surface contour dorsomedially is not straight and has a prominent, rounded ridge for the attachment of the dorsal ligament.

(9) Comparable proximodistal thickness of the central and third tarsal bones.

C. The Medial Oblique View

• Centering the MO view – The x-ray beam is centered at the central tarsal bone, and a horizontal beam is used that is described as a dorso45°lateral-plantaromedial oblique (Figure 10-6). The medial oblique is taken at 45° from the D-Pl plane. This obliquity highlights the medial region of the tarsus in the region where the cunean tendon passes obliquely over the tarsus to insert on MTIII and the first tarsal bone. This region must be examined carefully for radiographic signs of secondary joint disease and productive bony change in the attachment of the dorsal ligament on the medial aspect of the central and third tarsal bones and proximal MT III and MT II (Figure 10-7).

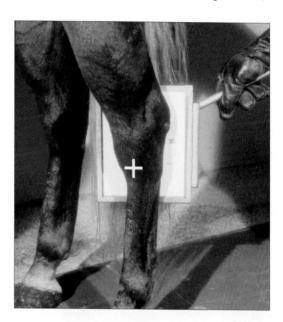

Figure 10-6. The medial oblique (MO) view is produced by an x-ray beam centered at the central tarsal bone and directed dorso45°lateral-plantaro-medial oblique.

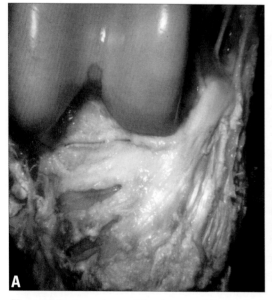

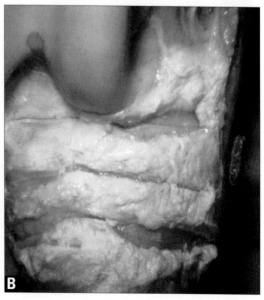

Figure 10-7. A specimen of the dorsum of the tarsus demonstrates the extensive dorsal ligament originating from the distal tuberosity of the talus **(A)**. Removal of the body of the dorsal ligament demonstrates its broad attachment on the central and third tarsal bones plus proximal MT III, and that the dorsolateral aspect of the DIT joint is more proximally located than the dorsomedial aspect **(B)**. This anatomical difference which can also be seen radiographically in Figure 10-3 results in a unique positional adjustment to produce the latero-medial and the lateral oblique views.

- Primary anatomical areas of the tarsus identified radiographically (Figure 10-8) with the MO view are:
  - Dorsomedial and plantarolateral surfaces, cortices, periarticular regions, and subchondral bone of the distal tibia, tarsus, and proximal metatarsus.
  - Medial ridge of the trochlea of the talus.
  - Lateral ridge of the trochlea of the talus.
  - Dorsum of the intermediate ridge of the tibia.
  - Proximal and distal tuberosities of the talus.
  - Coracoid process of the calcaneus.
  - Fourth tarsal bone, the head of MT IV, and plantar surface of lateral MT III.
  - Dorsomedial contour of the third tarsal bone which appears as a central prominence with a smooth periosteal surface.

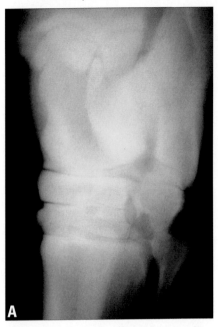 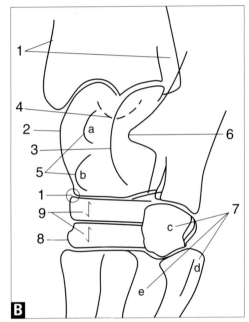

Figure 10-8. *The MO radiographic view **(A and B)** allows interpretation of:*
- *(1) Dorsomedial and plantarolateral surfaces, cortices, periarticular regions, and subchondral bone of the distal tibia, tarsus, and proximal metatarsus.*
- *(2) Medial ridge of the trochlea of the talus.*
- *(3) Lateral ridge of trochlea of the talus.*
- *(4) Dorsum of the intermediate ridge of the tibia.*
- *(5) Proximal (a) and distal (b) tuberosities of the talus.*
- *(6) Coracoid process of the calcaneus.*
- *(7) Fourth tarsal bone (c), the head of MT IV (d), and plantar surface of the lateral MT III (e).*
- *(8) Dorsomedial contour of the third tarsal bone appears as a central prominence with a smooth periosteal surface. This ridge should be examined carefully for evidence of productive bony change indicative of enthesophyte formation.*
- *(9) Comparable proximodistal thickness of the central and third tarsal bones.*

D. The Lateral Oblique View

- Centering the LO view – The x-ray beam is centered at the central tarsal bone and the direction is accurately described as plantaro 5°disto60°lateral-dorsoproximomedial oblique (Figure 10-9). The dorsolateral aspect of the DIT joint has a natural configuration different from that seen on the dorsal or dorsomedial aspect. To visualize the dorsolateral aspect of the DIT joint the x-ray beam must be angled 5° distal to proximal. The 60° lateral angulation from the plantar-dorsal plane highlights the dorsolateral area of the intertarsal joints where pathologic changes more commonly occur. The plantarodorsal direction of the x-ray beam is recommended rather than the dorsoplantar direction because it is more convenient for visualizing the anatomy of the tarsus.

Figure 10-9. *The lateral oblique (LO) view has compound angulation produced with an x-ray beam centered at the central tarsal bone and directed as a plantaro5°disto60°lateral-dorsoproximomedial oblique.*

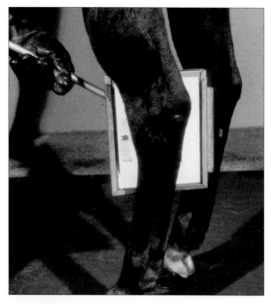

- Primary anatomical areas of the tarsus identified radiographically (Figure 10-10) with the LO view are:
  - Dorsolateral and plantaromedial surfaces, cortices, periarticular, and subchondral regions of the distal tibia, tarsus, and proximal metatarsus.
  - Dorsum of the intermediate ridge of the tibia.
  - Lateral ridge of the trochlea of the talus.
  - Medial ridge of the trochlea of the talus.
  - Surface and body of the sustentaculum tali.
  - Fused first and second tarsal bones and the head of MT II.

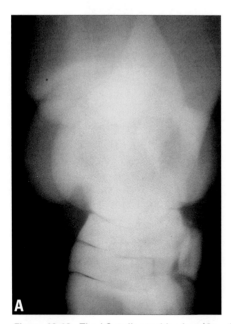

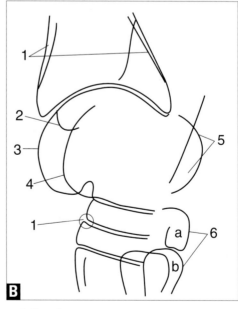

Figure 10-10. *The LO radiographic view (**A and B**) allows interpretation of:*
(1) The dorsolateral and plantaromedial surfaces, cortices, periarticular, and subchondral regions of the distal tibia, tarsus, and proximal metatarsus.
(2) Dorsum of the intermediate ridge of the tibia.
(3) Lateral ridge of the trochlea of the talus.
(4) Medial ridge of the trochlea of the talus.
(5) Surface and body of the sustentaculum tali.
(6) Fused first and second tarsal bones (a) and the head of MT II (b).

2. Special Radiographic Views of the Tarsus: Three

There are three views taken to supplement the routine examination of the tarsus. These are the flexed-plantaro75°proximal to the plantarodistal oblique (calcaneal skyline), the flexed-lateromedial (f-LM), and the flexed-dorso0°proximal-plantarodistal oblique (f-DPI). **As a general rule, the AEP should also take the similar special view of the opposite limb.** This approach is strongly recommended because the AEP is relatively unfamiliar with the radiographic anatomy, and the abnormal radiographic findings will be more easily recognized when a direct comparison can be made for differences. This latter reason is true because many abnormalities are either unilateral or differ in the degree of severity of the changes when bilateral.

  A. Flexed-Pl75°Pr-PlDiO or calcaneal skyline view - The indication for this view is to evaluate the tuber calcis, sustentaculum tali, medial ridge of the talus, and the tarsal groove (Figure 10-11). Different exposure times are required for this view dependent upon whether the tuber calcis or sustentaculum tali is to be evaluated. In practice, the tuber calcis exposure is routinely made unless a sustentacular lesion is suspected.

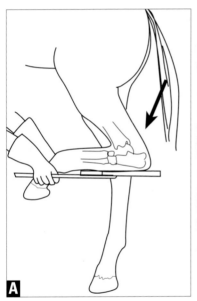
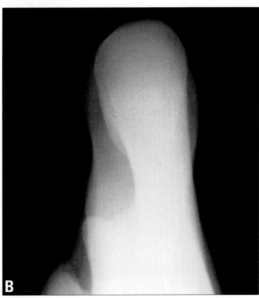
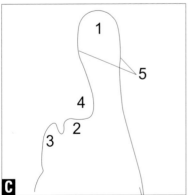

Figure 10-11. *The calcaneal skyline view is taken with the tarsus in a flexed position and the x-ray beam directed from the plantaroproximal to plantarodistal at a 75° proximal angulation **(A)**. This special view **(B and C)** is taken to evaluate the tuber calcis (1), sustentaculum tali (2), medial ridge of the talus (3), and the tarsal groove (4) for destructive lesions, fractures, and soft tissue density changes suspected or not seen with radiographic views of the routine examination. Productive bony response on the medial and/or lateral surface(s) of the tuber calcis is seen associated with bony change at the attachment of the superficial digital flexor tendon (5) as it forms the "calcanean cap."*

  B. Flexed-LM View – The indication for this view is to further evaluate the trochlea of the talus (Figure 10-12). The LM view allows the dorsum of the trochlea to be evaluated distally but the area of the trochlea articulating with the distal tibia seen on the LM cannot be evaluated completely. The flexed-LM permits this region of the trochlea to be better visualized and interpreted for contour abnormalities and density changes.

O'BRIEN'S RADIOLOGY FOR THE AMBULATORY EQUINE PRACTITIONER

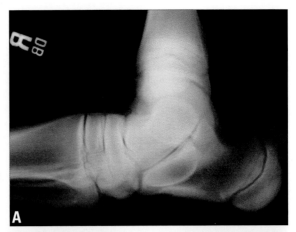

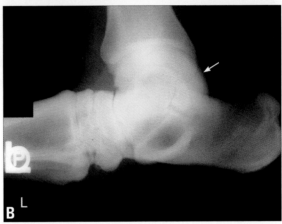

Figure 10-12. *In the foal the Flexed-LM is a special view that is valuable to evaluate the distal tibial physis and epiphysis, the physis and apophysis of the tuber calcis, and the subchondral bone of the tarsocrural joint (**A**). This view allows the trochlea of the talus to be evaluated at the normal weight-bearing region for contour abnormalities and density changes in the mature horse (**B**).*

C. **Flexed-DPI View** – The indication for this view is in the foal and younger horse. This view allows better assessment of the distal tibial epiphysis, lateral and medial malleoli, and the tarsocrural joint (Figure 10-13). In the mature horse, this view allows a more complete evaluation of the subchondral bone of the tarsocrural joint and the malleoli.

3. Exposure Factors

These tarsal projections can be produced with a portable x-ray machine, 400 speed imaging system, and a film-focal distance of 26 inches. The exposure factors for a mature, standard sized horse will vary depending on working conditions, but exposure times using 80kVp and 10 mA are given to serve as a reference point to be adjusted to one's working conditions.

- Dorsoplantar and the flexed-lateromedial views: 0.14 sec.
- Lateromedial and oblique views: 0.1 sec.
- Calcaneal skyline for tuber calcis: 0.1 sec.
- Calcaneal skyline for the sustentaculum: 0.14 sec.

An aluminum cassette holder is required to produce these views but a grid is not.

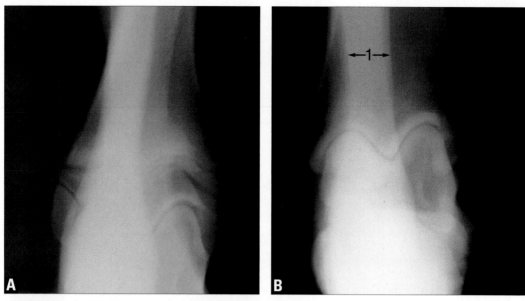

Figure 10-13. *The Flexed-dorsoplantar view is a special view taken more commonly in the foal and younger horse to evaluate the distal tibial epiphysis, growth plate of the lateral malleous and tarsocrural joint (**A**). This view is taken in the mature horse to evaluate the subchondral bone of the tarsocrural joint and the malleoli without the calcaneus superimposed (**B**). The Achilles tendon produces the uniform increased density with a sharply marginated axial border extending from the distal tibia over the lateral half of the talus (1).*

III. Interpretation of the Tarsus

As indicated by a general statement in the Introduction, abnormalities of the tarsus are classified into five diagnostic categories. The radiographic findings associated with each will be discussed.

1. Soft Tissue Swelling (STS) without Bony Changes

The first radiographic determinations to be made are whether STS is present and if the STS is confined to the joint capsule (intracapsular).

- Intracapsular STS at the tarsus is confined to the tarsocrural and proximal intertarsal joints.
- The distal intertarsal (DIT) and tarsometatarsal (TMT) joints have small dorsal volumes and tight joint capsules which cannot be identified radiographically as intracapsular distension.
- The intracapsular STS will be seen as an increased density with a dorsal convexity at the level of the dorsum of the talus and distal tibia (Figure 10-14). There will also be increased density plantar to the distal tibia, but this radiographic finding is more difficult to identify because it tends to be less sharply marginated.
- The clinical conditions compatible with intracapsular STS without bony changes are serous arthritis (bog spavin) and infectious arthritis. The history and clinical signs are important determinates of the cause.

The serous arthritis usually has a chronic history of the clinical problem, and the infectious arthritis is usually associated with an acute clinical problem and a greater degree of lameness. If the clinical history is compatible with a serous arthritis and the degree of STS is prominent, careful evaluation of the dorsal part of the intermediate ridge on the LM and LO oblique views for fragmentation should be done.

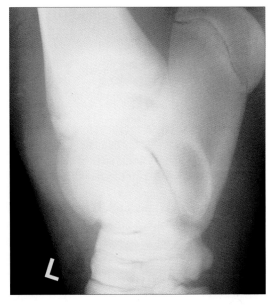

Extracapsular STS at the tarsus is more diffuse with loss of tissue planes extending proximally and distally. An evaluation of all four radiographic views reveals the STS is more restricted to one area than its opposite companion area, i.e., medial versus lateral or dorsomedial versus dorsolateral. Direct trauma, circulatory disorders, cellulitis, and bursitis are the usual differential diagnoses associated with extracapsular STS. Dystrophic calcification is occasionally seen with extracapsular STS (Figure 10-15). Corticosteroid injections administered for chronic lameness are often associated with calcification.

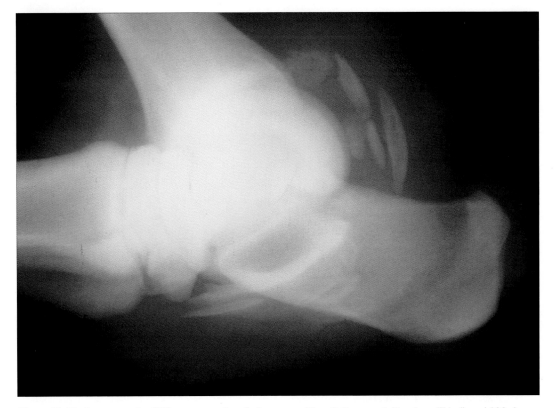

Figure 10-15. Extracapsular STS may occasionally be seen with soft tissue calcification. This flexed-LM shows how the calcification conforms to the tarsal sheath.

Radiographic Interpretation of the Tarsus

2. Secondary Joint Disease (Osteoarthritis or Spavin)

A. Introduction

The term "spavin" is commonly used with secondary joint disease (SJD) at the tarsus. Spavin is defined[1] as "In general, an exostosis, usually medial, of the equine tarsus, distal to the tibiotarsal articulation and often involving the metatarsus. It is classified as a blood, bog, or bone spavin."

Radiographically, blood spavin appears as an extracapsular STS on the dorsomedial aspect of the tarsus, bog spavin as an intracapsular STS at the tarsocrural joint, and bone spavin is an arthritis at the intertarsal and tarsometatarsal articulations. The bone spavin is commonly followed by exostosis and ankylosis, and is called a Jack spavin when there is a very large exostotic spavin.

B. Radiographic Signs of SJD of the Tarsus Seen on the LM and Oblique Views

The radiographic signs of SJD of the tarsus seen on the LM and oblique views include productive and destructive changes involving the periarticular and subchondral regions of the intertarsal (primarily the DIT joint) and tarsometatarsal joints (Figure 10-16). Periosteal productive changes are

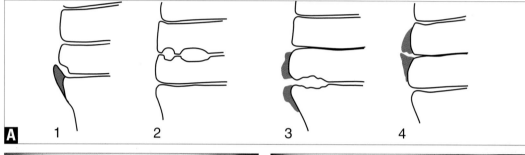

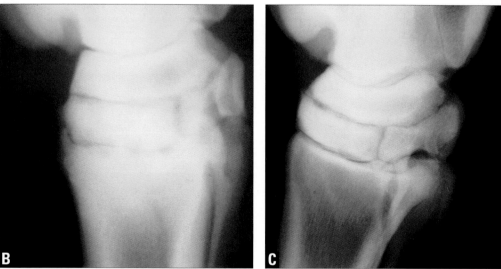

Figure 10-16. Radiographic findings of secondary joint disease (SJD) of the tarsus seen on the LM and oblique projections are schematically summarized *(A)*. Findings can occur either individually or collectively and include the following signs (radiographic examples of these signs are also demonstrated in *B and C*):
  (1) Periarticular productive and destructive changes at the dorsum of the intertarsal and tarsometatarsal (TMT) joints (B).
  (2) Decreased density in the subchondral bone dorsally varying in appearance from cystic to more generalized lucencies.
  (3) Irregularity to the subchondral bone and loss of the joint space width.
  (4) Periosteal productive change at the dorsum of the central and third tarsal bones (C) and the dorsoproximal third metatarsus.
  (5) Convex appearing dorsum to the central and third tarsal bones with loss of joint space (ankylosis) is seen in more chronic stages (see Figure 10-5D for diagnostic information).

[1] Dorland's Illustrated Medical Dictionary. W. B. Saunders Company, 24th Edition, p. 1141.

also seen dorsally in the areas of attachment of the dorsal ligament (see Figure 10-7) and the degree of these periosteal changes can be extensive leading to bridging across the joint producing extracapsular ankylosis. More commonly there is also intracapsular ankylosis of the involved joint secondary to articular cartilage and subchondral bony breakdown. The pathological changes described radiographically can be seen individually or collectively.

A radiographic finding that is seen approximately in the middle of the DIT and TMT joints is a focal lucency (Figure 10-17). The lucency at the level of the DIT joint tends to be cystic while at the tarsometatarsal joint the lucency appears more elongated in the dorsoplantar direction. However, the proximal part of the "cyst" at the DIT joint appears to be formed in the distal subchondral bone of the central tarsal bone, and the distal part of the "cyst" appears to be in the proximal subchondral bone of the third tarsal bone. These focal lucencies represent normal radiographic findings created by non-articular depressions in the respective bones and contain interosseous ligaments.

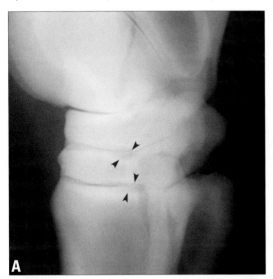 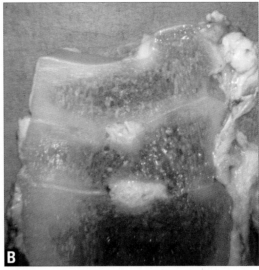

Figure 10-17. A focal lucency is seen near the middle of the DIT and TMT joints (arrows). The former tends to appear more cystic and latter more oblong **(A)**. These are normal findings resulting from non-articular depressions in the respective bones and these depressions contain interosseous ligaments **(B)**.

C. Radiographic Signs of SJD of the Tarsus Seen on the DPI View

The radiographic signs of SJD at the DIT joint seen on the DPI view are summarized schematically (Figure 10-18). The four radiographic findings are:

1. Narrowing or loss of joint space width.
2. Periarticular productive changes (osteophytes) medial and/or laterally.
3. Loss of subchondral bone of the distal central and proximal third tarsal bones creating a focally wide and more irregular appearing joint space.
4. Increased density (opacity) accompanying the joint space changes described in 3.

As demonstrated in Figure 10-2, joint space width of the intertarsal joints is influenced significantly by proximal angulation. The degree of proximal angulation is determined by the relationship of the head of MT IV and DIT joint. Loss of joint space width is a sign of SJD. This determination is made by comparing the widths of the proximal intertarsal (PIT), DIT, and TMT joints. The loss or narrowing of the DIT joint space with "normal" appearing widths to the PIT and TMT joint spaces is a significant finding. Loss or narrowing on all three joints is more likely to be artifactual. To more accurately interpret the loss or narrowing of all three joints, this three-joint comparison should also be done on the oblique views. Irregularity and decreased density to the subchondral bone at the DIT joint also indicates SJD. This finding usually is seen on the medial half of the DIT joint. Periarticular productive change at the DIT joint is more commonly seen medially on the DPI view. A periarticular osteophyte may be seen at the lateral aspect of the DIT joint appearing as a small overlapping "lip" of bone (figure 10-18C). This finding of SJD when originating from the distolateral central tarsal bone has been referred to as a "thoroughbred hook." A sclerotic stripe or band of increased density running parallel to the DIT joint space in the mid- to distal body of the central and the proximal- to mid body of the third tarsal bones often accompanies irregularity and decreased density to the subchondral bone of the DIT joint.. This finding results from the chronic productive change described previously for the LM view (Figure 10-16 A4).

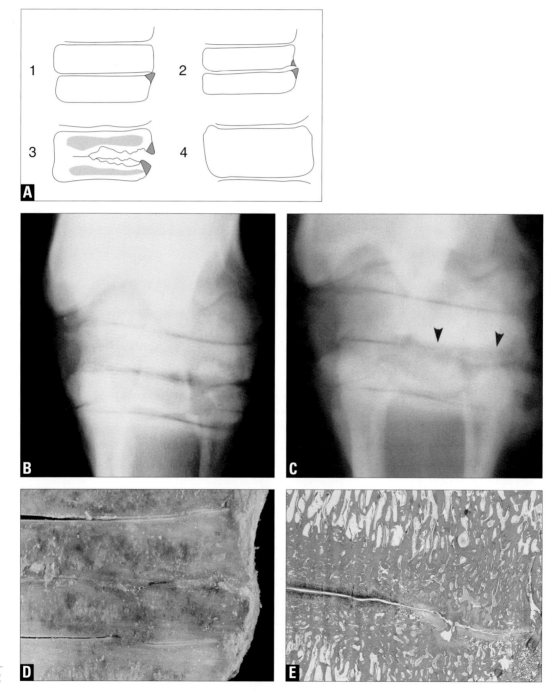

Figure 10-18. The radiographic findings of SJD of the DIT joint seen on the DPI projection are schematically summarized *(A)*. These findings can occur either individually or collectively and include the following signs (radiographic examples of these signs are also demonstrated in *B, C, and F*):

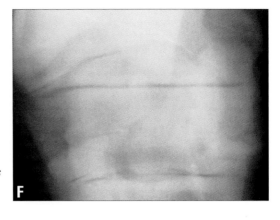

  (1) Periarticular osteophyte at the medial and/or lateral aspects of the DIT joint.
  (2) Irregularity and decreased density in the subchondral bone (B).
  (3) A sclerotic stripe of bone or increased density parallel to the DIT joint space (C). This finding is produced by the periosteal bony change on the dorsum of the central and third tarsal bones described in Figure 10-16.
  (4) Gross (D) and microscopic (E) appearance of loss of the medial joint space width. This determination is done radiographically by a comparison of the medial and lateral widths of the PIT, DIT, and TMT joints. The loss of all three or a tapering reduction in width from the PIT to TMT are usually positioning artifact, while the loss of the DIT and presence of the PIT and TMT indicates fusion (F).

3. Fractures

Tarsal fractures are relatively uncommon but when they are encountered, there seem to be four clinical presentations. The first is associated with a catastrophic injury resulting in non-weight bearing lameness and extensive STS. Complete fractures of the distal tibia, body of the talus, and body of the calcaneus are the most commonly seen with this clinical presentation. The second type of presentation is a mild to moderate degree of lameness and a minor degree of STS mainly at the level of the distal tarsus. Periarticular fractures of the dorsum of the central tarsal and third tarsal bones and dorsoproximal third metatarsus are most commonly seen with this clinical presentation (Figure 10-19). The third type of presentation is a mild to moderate degree of lameness and STS in the plantar region of the tarsus and the flexor tendon sheath. This clinical presentation is often associated with a fracture from the medial aspect of the sustentaculum tali (Figure 10-20). The calcaneal skyline view is a special radiographic projection indicated to evaluate the horse with these clinical findings. Finally, slab fractures of the central and third tarsal bones are seen with moderate to severe lameness and a history of an acute onset. The severity of lameness seems to be proportional to the degree of separation at the fracture seen radiographically. Incomplete slab fractures can be extremely difficult to identify radiographically during the acute phases. Scintigraphy has been utilized to supplement radiology in the diagnosis (Figure 10-21). If scintigraphy is not available, it is recommended the horse with clinical signs compatible with a slab fracture be referred to a facility with scintigraphy or restricted to a stall with a cross-tie and follow-up radiographs taken at 7-10 days.

The growth plate at the lateral malleolus is of importance radiographically because it is often confused* with a fracture because the AEP is unfamiliar with the presence in this anatomical structure and the appearance of a linear lucency running in an oblique plane to the subchondral surface of the distal tibia (Figure 10-22). A fracture of the lateral malleolus is usually identified as a displaced osseous body with an abnormal contour to the malleolus identifying the site of origin. The displacement results from the pulling of the lateral collateral ligament. The radiographic interpretation must determine if there is comminution of the fracture because comminution tends to make the surgical treatment more difficult.

*Remember, confusion can be eliminated or greatly decreased by taking a DPI view of the opposite tarsus!

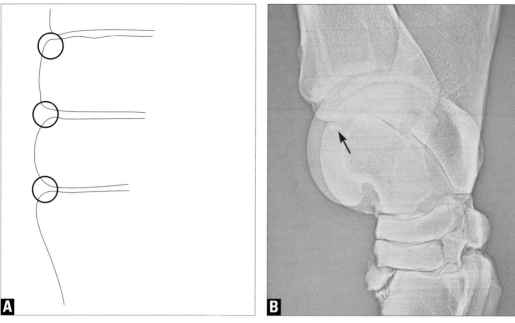

Figure 10-19. *Periarticular fractures in the tarsus commonly involve the dorsum of the central and third tarsal bones and the dorsoproximal MT III (A). These fractures often are seen in the horse with a mild to moderate degree of lameness and a limited degree of STS. They can vary from small, chip fractures, to large corner fractures (B). The large corner fracture was identified using xeroradiography in a racing thoroughbred at the racetrack. An OCD lesion of the intermediate ridge of the distal tibia is seen in this horse with a fracture.*

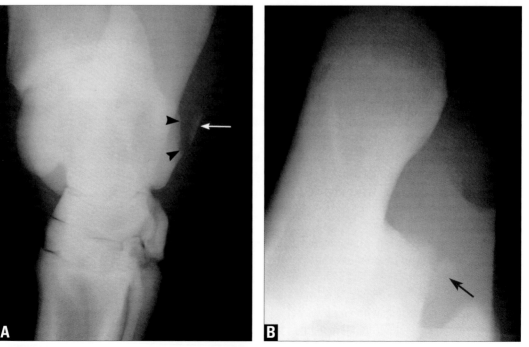

Figure 10-20. *Superficial sustentacular fractures (arrow) are usually seen originating from the medial aspect of the sustentaculum tali (arrowheads) associated with plantar extracapsular soft tissue swelling and mild to moderate degree of lameness (A). A calcaneal skyline view is indicated for a more complete radiographic evaluation (B).*

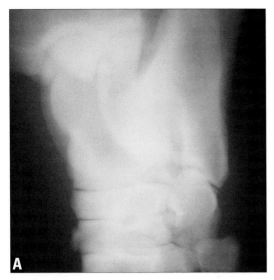

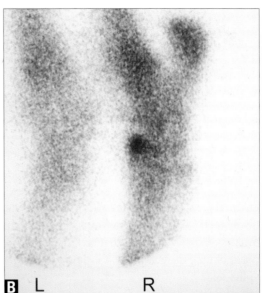

Figure 10-21. An incomplete slab fracture of the central and/or third tarsal bones may not be visible radiographically in horses with acute onset of a severe degree of lameness **(A)**. Nuclear medical imaging **(B)** revealed a significant amount of isotopic uptake in right tarsus when compared to the left tarsus. The uptake in the right image in the region of the central tarsal bone is compatible with a fracture and occurred several days before a radiographic diagnosis could be made **(C)**. Nuclear medical imaging is extremely valuable in evaluating hind limb lameness in horses. Its common role is to identify locations where a radiographic examination should be taken to provide more specificity to a diagnosis.

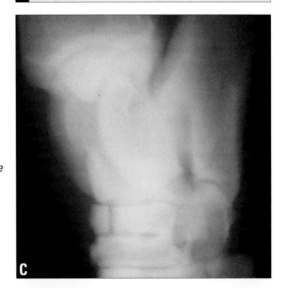

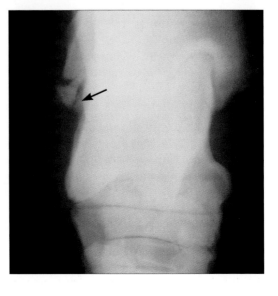

Figure 10-22. The growth plate of the lateral malleolus is identified as an oblique linear lucency extending from the subchondral surface of the distolateral tibia (see Figure 10-13A). A fracture of the lateral malleolus can usually be identified as a displaced fragment of bone caused by the pull of the lateral collateral ligament, but the fracture must be carefully evaluated radiographically for comminution which has important surgical implications.

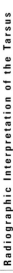

4. Infection

The radiographic interpretation of bone and joint infection in the horse was presented in Chapter 3. Unique features of this topic as it relates to the radiographic interpretation of the tarsus will be emphasized here. There are two clinical situations deserving consideration – one in the immature and one in the mature horse.

A. Septic Physitis and Osteomyelitis in the Immature Horse

The growth plates in the tarsal region of radiographic interest are at the distal tibia, tuber calcis, and the lateral malleolus. Infection at the distal tibial and tuber calcis growth plates is identified radiographically as a destructive process. This process commonly extends into the adjacent epiphysis and apophysis, respectively, and may lead to pathological fractures resulting in a guarded prognosis. The flexed-dorsoplantar view is important to evaluate the distal epiphysis of the distal tibia when trauma (fracture) or infection is suspected. This view permits better evaluation of the proximal to distal thickness and shape. The shape of this thin epiphysis is a result of the proximal contour created by the physis and distal contour conforming to the trochlea of the talus.

B. Tarsal Osteomyelitis in the Mature Horse

The incidence of bone and joint infections of the tarsus in the mature horse tends to be low but when seen the causes are often iatrogenic or secondary to severe trauma. Osteomyelitis of the tuber calcis is unique radiographically because of its location and radiographic appearance. The radiographic signs include:

1. Soft tissue swelling over the tuber calcis.
2. Focal lucency in the bony surface that is difficult to identify on the LM and oblique views in the early stages because the bony contour is recessed.
3. Increased density to the body of the tuber calcis is associated with chronicity.

A diagnosis of osteomyelitis is suspected based on the clinical signs and radiographic findings, but these radiographic findings are difficult to identify. Under these circumstances, the AEP should ask what can be done to assist in the radiographic evaluation. The answer is a special radiographic examination, i.e., skyline of the calcaneus (Figure 10-23). It is important to emphasize that a skyline view of the opposite calcaneus should be taken for comparison to assist in the interpretation by the AEP.

5. Developmental Orthopedic Disease (DOD)

The intermediate ridge of the tibia and the ridges of the talus are the specific locations for OCD in the tarsus. Developmental disease is seen at the dorsum of the central and third tarsal bones. **A bilateral radiographic examination should be taken routinely for evaluation of DOD of the tarsus.**

A. OCD of the Intermediate Ridge of the Tibia

Intermediate ridge lesions are identified at a specific anatomical location at the dorsum of this ridge. These lesions may be seen on the LM projection but they are best visualized on the lateral oblique view as either a single or multiple osseous bodies that may or may not be displaced from the site. The site of origin is identified as an abnormal contour to the dorsum of the intermediate ridge (Figure 10-24). These lesions can be present without producing clinical signs. The need for surgical removal is usually correlated to the degree of clinical lameness and presence of intracapsular distension of the tarsocrural joint.

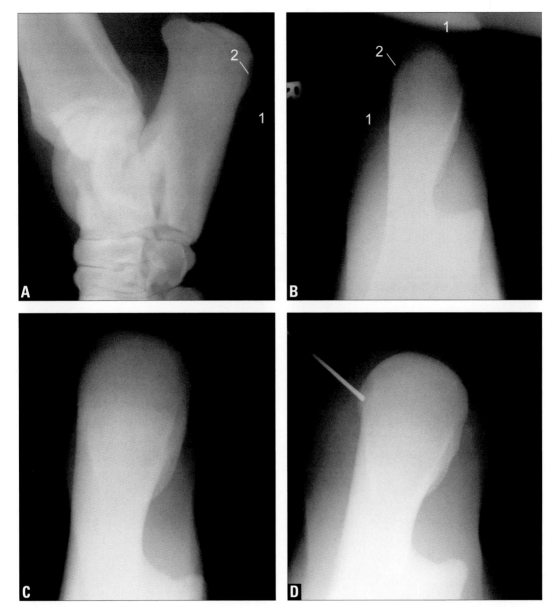

Figure 10-23. Osteomyelitis of the tuber calcis in the early stages is a difficult radiographic diagnosis which can be demonstrated in a horse with swelling and a draining track at the right tuber calcis. The radiographic signs are:
(1) Soft tissue swelling over the tuber calcis.
(2) Focal surface lucency in the calcaneus that is difficult to identify is suspected with routine radiographic views **(A)**.
(3) In the chronic stages, an increased density to body of the tuber calcis secondary to periosteal reaction on the medial and lateral surfaces at the insertion of the superficial digital flexor tendon.
(4) A calcaneal skyline is indicated to evaluate this area **(B)**. A faint lucency of the lateral surface of the right tuber calcis (2) again is suspected. A comparison skyline of the left **(C)** was taken that demonstrated normal soft tissue density and thickness plus a smooth contour with uniform underlying bony density to the lateral aspect of the tuber calcis. This comparison provides a basis for more confidence in the suspected lucency in the right being a significant bony change. Another skyline was taken with a metal probe in the draining track to confirm communication to the bone at the location where the suspected changes were identified **(D)**. A medial oblique view was also taken (orthogonal view principle) with the probe to permit the confirmation.

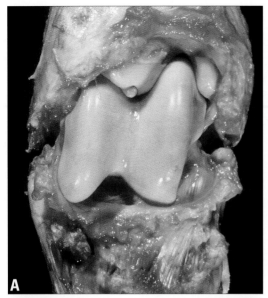

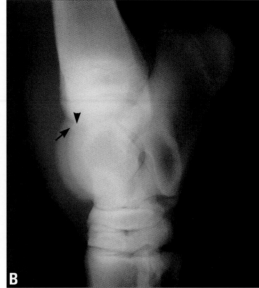

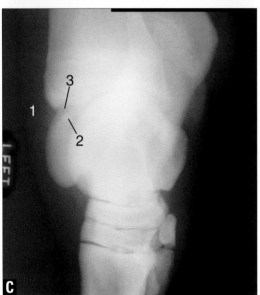

Figure 10-24. *Osteochondrosis of the intermediate ridge of the tibia occurs at a specific location on the dorsal aspect (**A**). This lesion (arrowhead) can be seen on the LM (**B**) but is best visualized on the LO (**C**). The radiographic signs include: intracapsular STS (1), osseous body at the dorsum of the intermediate ridge (2), and a contour defect in intermediate ridge (3). However, variation in number, size, and degree of displacement of the osseous body can be seen in patients with this condition. This radiographic lesion may be an incidental finding (see Figure 10-19B). Intracapsular STS is a good indication of the clinical significance of this radiographic finding and the need for surgical removal.*

B. OCD of the Ridge of the Trochlea of the Talus

This OCD lesion can be identified with intracapsular STS as an abnormal contour at the mid-dorsal aspect of the ridge, and the underlying bone is usually less dense when the lesion is active (Figure 10-25). Fragments may be displaced distally or associated with the lesion and there may be undermining of the proximal or distal margins at the site of origin of a lesion. Another radiographic presentation with OCD can occur as a growth impairment of a ridge of the talus where the subchondral bone did not break down. Healing of this type of lesion can result in a focal region of flattening of the ridge identified as an abnormal contour with normal appearing underlying subchondral bone (Figure 10-26). This change is a result of a past temporary growth impairment without breakdown of the subchondral bone, and it is usually not associated with clinical signs of lameness. Identification of this bony change is important for purchase examinations.

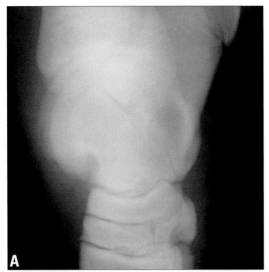

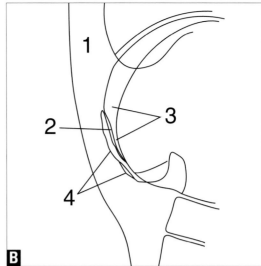

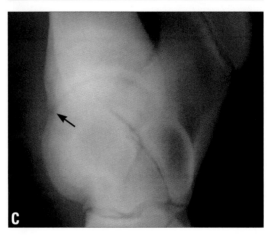

Figure 10-25. *OCD of the trochlea of the talus is usually seen at the mid-dorsal aspect of the lateral ridge* *(A)*. *A line drawing of* *(A)* *identifying abnormal radiographic findings* *(B)*. *The radiographic findings are: intracapsular STS (1), an abnormal contour to the lateral ridge (2), decreased density to the subchondral bone surrounded by increased bony density (3), superficial fragmentation associated with the other bony changes (4), or displaced distally. These findings were identified on the LM view* *(C)* *during a six-week re-examination but another contour abnormality can be seen in the* medial *ridge (arrow).*

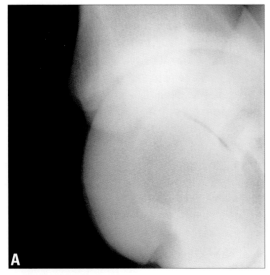

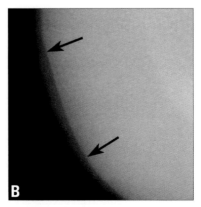

Figure 10-26. *Another radiographic manisfestation of osteochondrosis of the trochlear ridge of the talus is a focally flat appearance to the contour* *(A)*. *A slightly magnified image* *(B)* *of the trochlear ridges reveals this abnormal contour (arrows) contrasted to the normal contour of the other trochlear ridge of the talus. The lesion was localized to the lateral ridge using the oblique views. The underlying bone appeared normal for density and trabecular structure.*

A separate osseous body with a loss of the normal contour of the distal part of the lateral ridge of the talus has been described as an OCD. This lesion is more likely a fracture produced by direct trauma to this exposed lateral area (Figure 10-27). The appearance of a sharply marginated site of origin with normal bone density occurring at the distal aspect of the lateral ridge are the keys to diagnosing the lesion as a fracture.

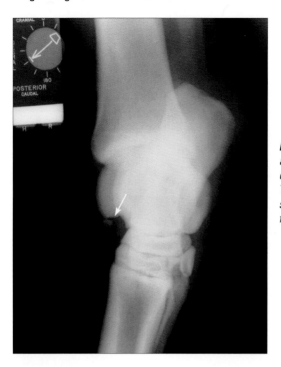

Figure 10-27. *A separate osseous body from the distal aspect of the lateral ridge of the talus resulting from direct traum to this expose area of the talus is seen. The site of origin of the fracture fragment (arrow) is sharply defined compatible with an acute complete fracture.*

C. Absence of Normal Trabecular Pattern at the Dorsum of the Central and/or Third Tarsal Bones

This condition has been referred to as "aseptic necrosis" of the central and/or third tarsal bones in the foal. Collapse of the third and/or central tarsal bones in the foal can result in abnormal contour to the tarsus (sickle hock) on the clinical examination. The radiographic findings include either a lack of or abnormal ossification of the central and/or third tarsal bone dorsally (Figure 10-28). Partially ossified fragmentation with dorsal displacement and subluxation of the PIT joint characterized by plantar displacement of the talus may be seen. The prognosis for a clinically sound horse is poor when these radiographic signs are present, but there are various degrees of ossification abnormalities.

A mild degree of this abnormal developmental process can be seen resulting in a reduction in the proximal to distal thickness of a tarsal bone (Figure 10-29). **A bilateral radiographic examination should be taken routinely for evaluation of developmental disorders of the tarsal bones.** This size reduction may be unilateral or bilateral, but when unilateral a comparison to the normal tarsus reveals angulation with subchondral sclerosis of the involved bone(s). Secondary joint disease commonly results in the tarsus as the horse develops (Figure 10-30). Differentiating a developmental disorder with secondary joint disease from a secondary joint disease from other causes requires careful radiographic evaluation of the thickness and shape of the tarsal bones (Figure 10-31). Chronic deformation with a proximal-to-distal narrowing of a tarsal bone identifies the underlying problem as a developmental disorder.

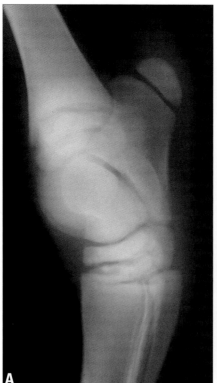

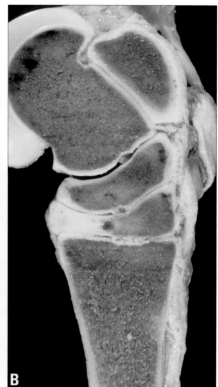

Figure 10-28. *A developmental disorder is seen in the ossification of the central and/or third tarsal bones **(A)**. Radiographic signs include: delayed ossification in the dorsum of these bones, collapse of these bones, and fragmentation with dorsal displacement of ossified and non-ossified fragments. The gross **(B)** and macroradiographic **(C)** appearances of bones with these changes are demonstrated.*

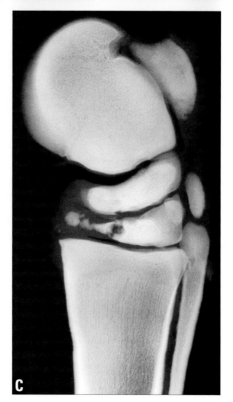

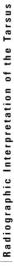

Radiographic Interpretation of the Tarsus

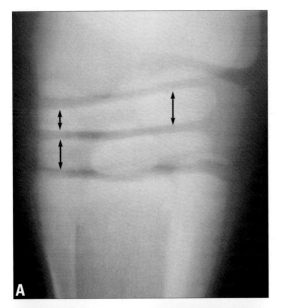

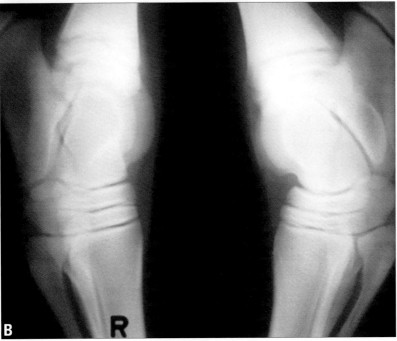

Figure 10-29. *A milder degree of developmental orthopedic disease of the central and/or third tarsal bones can be identified radiographically by a height differential between the medial and lateral halves of these bones, i.e., medial is less, and increased in density (A). Comparison LM radiographs of the left and right tarsi confirm these findings in the left tarsus to involve both the central and third tarsal bones (B).*

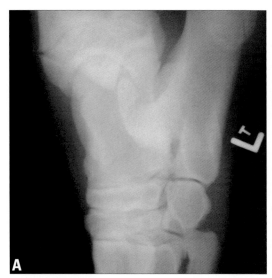

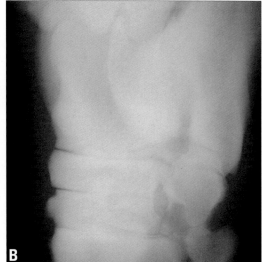

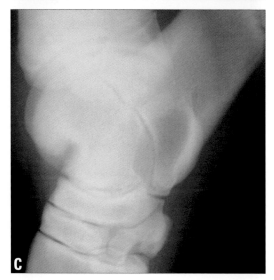

Figure 10-30. *As the foal in Figure 10-29 with a milder degree of developmental abnormality of primarily the central tarsal bone grew, the residium of this disorder was identified on the MO view by the radiographic signs of a reduced proximal-to-distal thickness of the medial part of the central tarsal bone and subchondral sclerosis (A). These signs are evident when compared to an adult horse where the normal thickness of the central and third tarsal bones are comparable (B). Radiographic signs of secondary joint disease at the dorsum of both intertarsal joints were also seen at the 10-month follow-up examination (C).*

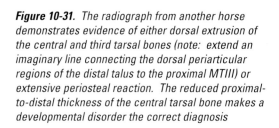

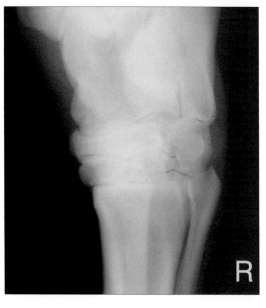

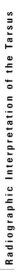

Figure 10-31. *The radiograph from another horse demonstrates evidence of either dorsal extrusion of the central and third tarsal bones (note: extend an imaginary line connecting the dorsal periarticular regions of the distal talus to the proximal MTIII) or extensive periosteal reaction. The reduced proximal-to-distal thickness of the central tarsal bone makes a developmental disorder the correct diagnosis*

NOTES

NOTES

NOTES

Chapter 11

Radiographic Interpretation of the Stifle and Proximal Tibia

I. Radiography

The routine radiographic examination of the stifle joint in the standing horse includes a latero-medial (LM), caudocranial (CC), and lateral oblique (caudo60°lateral-craniomedial oblique) projections. A medial oblique view is not included in the routine radiographic examination of the stifle. The AEP needs the following equipment to produce a diagnostic quality examination:

- X-ray unit capable of producing 90kVp and 10 mA exposures.
- Imaging system that has 400 speed. Rare earth screens and corresponding film in 14" x 17" cassettes are highly recommended.
- Aluminum cassette holder.
- Light beam collimator is very beneficial.
- A grid may be indicated due to the soft tissue thickness at the stifle, but it is not practical for the AEP because the exposure times required for a grid technique are greatly increased (2-4 times) and it would make positioning the cassette more difficult.

1. Views of the Routine Stifle Examination: Three
A. Caudocranial (CC) View

This view is exposed with the x-ray machine behind the horse and the cassette held cranially against the patella (Figure 11-1). Elevation of the ipsilateral front foot is indicated to aid in positioning the cassette in the flank region. The beam is centered at the soft tissue indentation at midline and directed horizontally or 5° downward, i.e., caudo5°proximal-craniodistal oblique. This angulation allows the intercondylar region of the femur to be seen more clearly. The CC view allows the distal femur, femorotibial joint spaces, and proximal tibia to be evaluated (Figure 11-2). If the distal femur is underexposed, a second CC view with an increased technique is indicated.

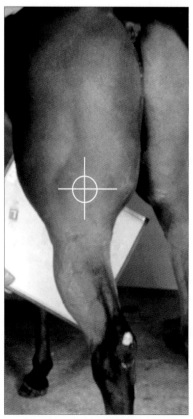

Figure 11-1. *The caudocranial view (CC) is produced with an x-ray beam centered on midline and perpendicular to the level of the femorotibial joint (marker).*

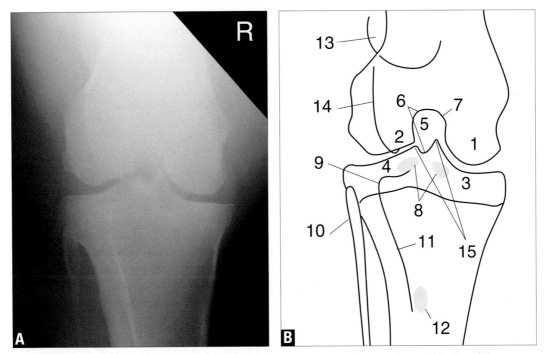

Figure 11-2. Radiograph of the CC view of a mature Quarter Horse stifle without abnormal findings **(A)**. A line drawing of **(A)** identifying anatomical structures of importance **(B)**.

1. Medial femoral condyle
2. Lateral femoral condyle
3. Medial tibial condyle
4. Lateral tibial condyle
5. Intercondylar fossa of the femur
6. Areas of attachment of the cranial cruciate ligament
7. Area of attachment of the caudal cruciate ligament
8. Areas of attachment for the cranial ligaments of the menisci
9. Tibial tuberosity
10. Fibula
11. Tibial crest
12. Attachment site for the semitendinosus tendon
13. Patella
14. Lateral ridge of the trochlea of the femur
15. Intercondylar eminences: medial (spine) and lateral

B. Lateromedial View

The cassette must be carefully placed medial to the stifle into the flank region. Elevation of the ipsilateral front foot is recommended to aid in this positioning. The x-ray beam is directed horizontally and centered caudodistal to the apex of the patella (Figure 11-3). The radiograph produced allows the cranial and caudal aspects of the distal femur, proximal tibia, and patella to be evaluated (Figure 11-4).

Another LM view may be included in the routine stifle examination. This view is indicated when the patient has an effusion of the femoropatellar joint. This LM view is centered on the patella and is taken with a reduced technique using a smaller (8" x 10") cassette. This optional radiograph is taken to evaluate the patella and the femoropatellar articulation in greater detail.

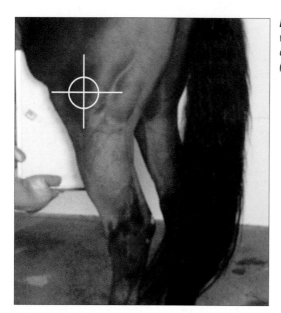

Figure 11-3. *The lateromedial view (LM) is produced with an x-ray beam centered caudodistal to the apex of the patella and horizontal to the femorotibial joint (marker).*

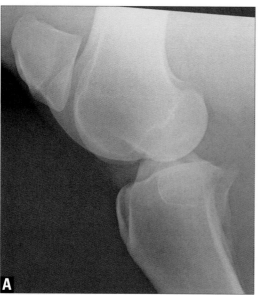

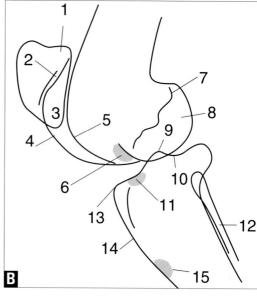

A **B**

Figure 11-4. *LM radiograph of a mature Thoroughbred without abnormal findings **(A)**. A line drawing of (A) identifying anatomical structures of importance **(B)**.*

1. *Base of patella*
2. *Medial femoropatellar articulation*
3. *Apex of patella*
4. *Medial ridge of the femoral trochlea*
5. *Lateral ridge of the femoral trochlea*
6. *Area of the extensor fossa*
7. *Distal femoral physeal scar*
8. *Femoral condyles*
9. *Tibial spine (medial intercondylar eminence)*
10. *Tibial condyle*
11. *Area of attachment for the cranial ligaments of the menisci*
12. *Fibula*
13. *Tibial tuberosity*
14. *Tibial crest*
15. *Area of attachment for the tendon of semitendinosus muscle*

C. Lateral Oblique View

The LO is produced with an x-ray beam parallel to the ground from the caudo60°lateral to cranio-medial direction. The beam is centered at the caudal aspect of the intercondylar region (Figure 11-5). The LO view allows the lateral ridge of the trochlea of the femur and the medial femoral condyle to be evaluated complementing interpretation of these anatomical areas on the LM and CC views (Figure 11-6). This view is extremely important in large breeds for evaluating the medial femoral condyle because the CC view may be underexposed as a result of equipment limitations of the AEP.

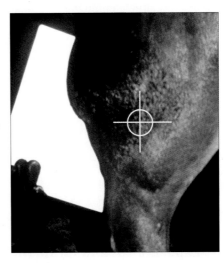

Figure 11-5. The lateral oblique view (LO) is produced with an x-ray beam directed horizontal to the femorotibial joint from the caudolateral to craniomedial direction. The angulation is 60° from the caudocranial plane.

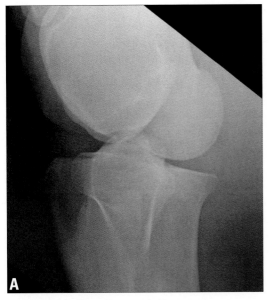

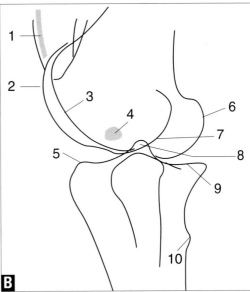

Figure 11-6. Radiograph of the LO projection of a mature Thoroughbred without abnormalities (**A**). A line drawing of (A) identifying anatomical structures of importance (**B**).
1. Attachment site for the biceps femoris and lateral patellar ligament
2. Lateral ridge of the femoral trochlea
3. Medial ridge of the femoral trochlea
4. Area of the extensor fossa
5. Tibial tuberosity
6. Medial femoral condyle
7. Lateral femoral condyle
8. Spine of the tibia
9. Medial condyle of the tibia
10. Tubercle

2. Special Radiographic Views of the Stifle

There are **two** views of the equine stifle that are taken to supplement the routine stifle radiographic examination. These include the patellar skyline (flexed-cranio85°proximal to craniodistal oblique) and the flexed-lateromedial (f-LM).

A. Patellar Skyline View

This view is taken with the stifle fully flexed and the tarsus either flexed or fully extended. The x-ray beam is directed from the region abaxial to the lumbar spine toward the cassette positioned against the tibia. The cassette must extend cranially to allow the silhouette of the patella to be captured on the radiograph (Figure 11-7). The radiograph produced allows the patella, femoropatellar joint, and trochlea of the femur to be evaluated (Figure 11-8). This special view is valuable to diagnose patellar fractures, osteochrondrosis, and secondary joint disease of the femoropatellar joint.

B. Flexed-Lateromedial View

The flexed-LM of the equine stifle is infrequently taken. The f-LM is indicated when craniocaudal instability from the rupture of the cruciate ligament is suspected and to evaluate the tibial plateau for an avulsion fracture or superficial lucencies associated with ligamentous injury at the bony surface. These surface lucencies are usually associated with the cranial ligaments of the menisci and occur more frequently medially than laterally.

3. Exposure Factors for Radiography of the Stifle

The AEP can produce stifle radiographs of diagnostic quality with an x-ray machine capable of producing 90kVp and 10mA. The focal-film distance is 26 inches and a 400-speed imaging system is required. The exposure time for the LM, LO, and patellar skyline views is approximately 0.2-0.4 seconds. The exposure time for the CC view is approximately double (0.4-0.8 seconds).

4. Chemical Restraint for Stifle Radiography

Sedation for the radiographic examination of the stifle is a requirement even though some older horses may be examined without it. The potential for injury when doing stifle radiography is too great not to utilize sedation.

The health related contra-indications for sedation of the equine patient must be carefully evaluated before administering any drug. Variation in the drug and dosage used depends on the nature of the horse and the duration of the sedation required. In our radiography practice, three intra-venous drugs are used to do stifle radiography. The demeanor of the horse and the anticipated duration of the examination are important variables in the consideration of which drugs should be used.

A. Short-term Sedation: Xylazine hydrochloride* provides approximately 15-20 minutes of sedation when administered at 0.3-0.4 mg/kg (approximately 150-200 mg/500 kg horse). Butorphanol tartrate** at 0.01 mg/kg or 5 mg/500 kg horse is sometimes added if there is a need to "plant the feet."

B. Longer-term Sedation: Detomidine hydrochloride*** provides approximately 30-40 minutes of sedation when administered at 0.01 mg/kg (approximately 5 mg/500 kg horse).

These dosages and drugs are guidelines for sedating the mature, healthy horse for stifle radiography.

* TranquiVed; VedCo. Inc.St. Joseph, MO 64507. ** Torbugesic. FortDodge Animal Health. Fort Dodge, Iowa, 50501. *** Dormosedan. Pfizer Animal Health. Exton, PA 19341.

Figure 11-7. *The patellar skyline view is taken with the stifle fully flexed. The cassette is placed cranially so the silhouette of the patella will be positioned completely on the radiograph.*

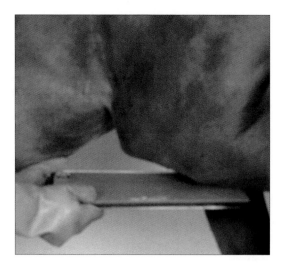

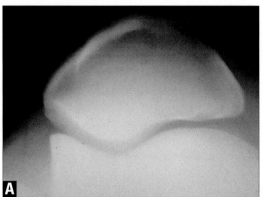

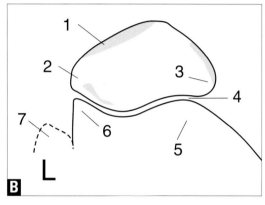

Figure 11-8. *The patellar skyline view of a mature Thoroughbred without radiographic abnormalities (**A**). A line drawing of (A) identifying anatomical structures of importance (**B**).*

1. Attachment area for the biceps femoris and the lateral patellar ligament
2. Lateral angle of the patella
3. Medial angle of the patella
4. Femoropatellar articulation
5. Medial ridge of the femoral trochlea
6. Lateral ridge of the femoral trochlea
7. Tibial tuberosity

II. Interpretation

There are four major abnormal radiographic signs associated with most of the conditions of the equine stifle. These signs are:

*   **Abnormal contour to the subchondral bone of the joint.**
*   **Density change in the subchondral bone. These density changes may be decreased, increased, or both.**
*   **Radiodense bodies associated with the areas of contour and density changes.**
*   **Periosteal reaction and signs of secondary joint disease including narrowing of the joint space, periarticular remodeling, and subchondral density changes.**

Interpretation of the stifle examination will be summarized by relating the anatomical regions seen on each radiographic view to these radiographic signs. The radiographic signs will then be correlated to Radiographic Conclusions/Impressions.

1. LM View: Radiographic Signs Associated with Anatomical Areas

The following anatomical areas are the locations where most radiographic abnormalities are seen on the LM view (Figure 11-9):

A. Trochlea Ridges of the Femur

    1) Abnormal contour to the lateral (Figures 11-10 and 11-11), medial, or both trochlear ridges (Figure 11-12).

    2) Underlying subchondral lucency.

    3) Sclerosis tends to surround the lucency.

    4) Radiodense body/bodies in the area of the abnormal contour or displaced distally.

Radiographic Conclusions/Impressions

- Osteochondrosis: Signs 1, 2, and 3
- Osteochondritis dissecans: Signs 1-4

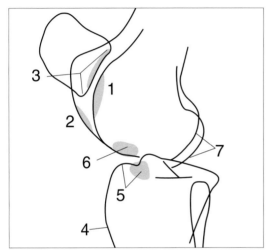

Figure 11-9. There are seven anatomical sites where most of the abnormal radiographic signs will be identified on the LM view. These sites are demonstrated schematically.

    1. Lateral ridge of the femoral trochlea
    2. Medial ridge of the femoral trochlea
    3. Periarticular and subchondral areas of the patella
    4. Tibial crest
    5. Tibial plateau and area of attachment of the cranial ligaments of the menisci (shaded area)
    6. Extensor fossa
    7. Femoral condyles

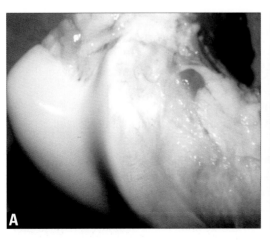

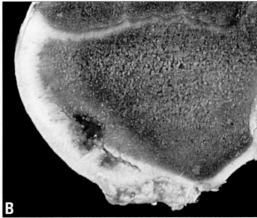

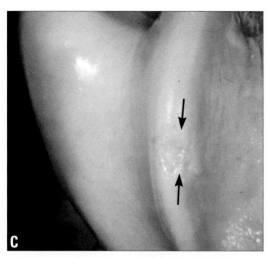

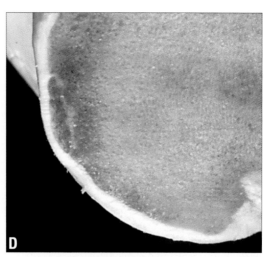

Figure 11-10. Gross pathology specimens of osteochondrosis of the lateral ridge of the femoral trochlea provides a greater understanding of the radiographic signs of this condition. This is a developmental orthopedic disease occurring from the interruption of the ossification process of the lateral ridge which is demonstrated with specimens from a yearling Quarter Horse. The articular cartilage appears normal **(A)** but there is extensive underlying change **(B)**. In the chronic stages of this developmental disease the gross lesions (arrows) may be focal **(C)** or extensive **(D)** resulting in variation in the appearance of the radiographic signs.

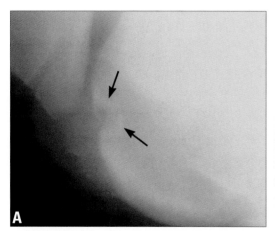

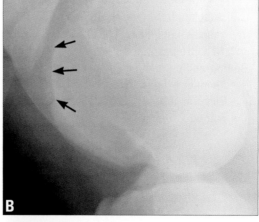

Figure 11-11. Osteochondrosis of the lateral ridge of the femoral trochlea is a common cause of femoropatellar joint effusion. The lesion is identified by three radiographic signs including contour abnormality, subchondral density change, and fragmentation (i.e., osteochondrosis dissecans). The lesion can vary in radiographic appearance from primarily a focal cystic lesion **(A)** with a minor degree of surrounding sclerosis (arrows), to a major contour abnormality (flattening) with a minor degree of density change **(B)**, to a major contour defect (1), deep subchondral lucency (2) with surrounding sclerosis (3) plus evidence of radiodense bodies (4) **(C)**.

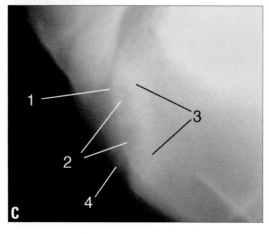

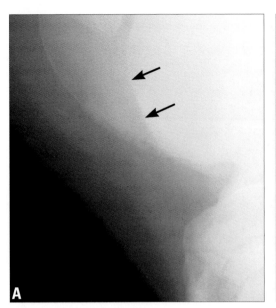
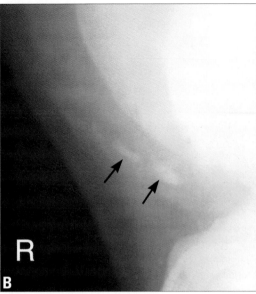

Figure 11-12. The radiographic signs of osteochondrosis of the medial ridge of the femoral trochlea **(A)** as compared to the lateral ridge are more subtle, superficial, and commonly seen occurring with a lateral ridge lesion (arrows). Displaced fragments from the primary lesion are commonly seen craniodistally (arrows) and it is fairly common for the fragment to embed within the synovium and increase in size with chronicity **(B)**.

B. Patella

1) Periarticular productive change at the apex or less commonly at the base.
2) Subchondral lucency in the mid-portion with surrounding sclerosis and periarticular remodeling (Figure 11-13).
3) Bony fragment at the apex or medial angle.

Radiographic Conclusions/Impressions

- Secondary joint disease: Sign 1
- Osteochondrosis: Signs 1 and 2
- Fracture: Sign 3

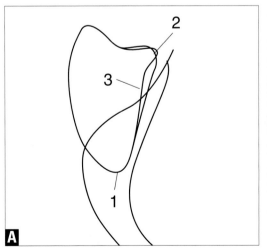
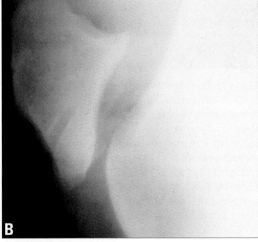

Figure 11-13. The locations for radiographic signs of abnormalities of the periarticular and articular areas of the patella seen on the LM view **(A)** are the apex (1), base (2), and subchondral bone (3). A ten-year old horse had radiographic signs of periarticular productive change at the base and apex with subchondral lucency and sclerosis in the mid-portion compatible with a diagnosis of severe secondary joint disease **(B)**.

C. Tibial Crest

1) Bony change to a focal region at the tibial crest centered approximately 11 cm distal to the tibial tuberosity (Figure 11-14).
   - Periosteal productive change
   - Decreased cortical density in this focal area
2) Abnormal contour with area.
3) Lucent linear line parallel to the cortical surface (uncommon).
4) Dense body at the cortical surface (uncommon).

Radiographic Conclusions/Impressions

- Enthesophytosis and/or an avulsion fracture at the site of insertion of the tendon of the semitendinosus on the tibial crest: Signs 1-4.

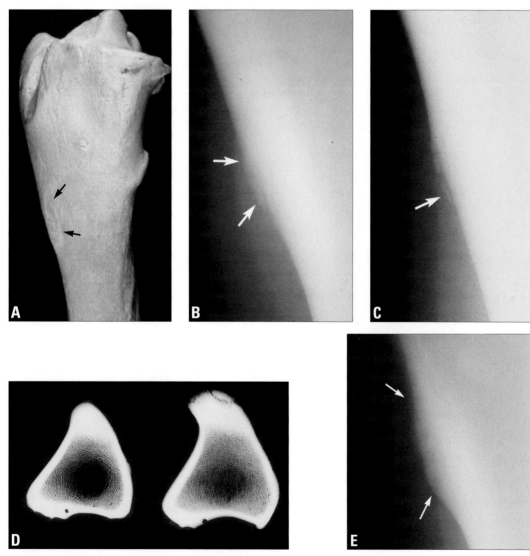

Figure 11-14. *Bony changes at the attachment of the tendon of the semitendinosus muscle on the tibia occur at a specific location on the tibial crest approximately 11 cm distal to the tibial tuberosity **(A)**. The early radiographic signs of a lesion at this location are a periosteal productive change and a superficial decreased cortical density **(B)**. An avulsion fracture (arrow) may be identified in the subacute stages **(C)**. Radiographs of bone specimens demonstrate the normal tibial crest and one with an avulsion fracture with extensive bony remodeling **(D)**. A chronic lesion can be identified as a contour abnormality appearing as a dorsal convexity **(E)**. The radiographic identification of bony change at this specific location must be followed with a radiographic examination of this area on the opposite tibia and a careful clinical examination of the area.*

D. Tibial Plateau and Extensor Fossa

1) Increased lucency in the cranial region of the tibial plateau (Figure 11-15).
2) A rim of sclerosis surrounding the lucency.
3) Increased lucency in the distal femur at the extensor fossa.

Radiographic Conclusions/Impressions

- The changes in the cranial tibial plateau result from fibro-osseous remodeling at the insertion of the cranial ligaments of the menisci. The medial cranial meniscal ligament is more commonly involved: Signs 1 and 2
- The change in the extensor fossa is secondary to fibro-osseous remodeling at the origin of the long digital extensor and peroneus tertius tendons: Sign 3

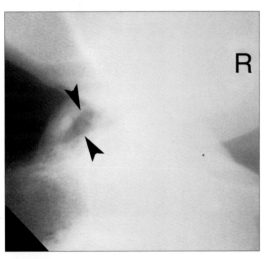

Figure 11-15. Enthesophyte formation associated with fibro-osseous damage at the attachment of the cranial ligament of the meniscus is identified radiographically on the LM view by a focal lucency (arrowheads) at the cranial aspect of the tibial plateau.

2. Caudocranial View: Radiographic Signs Associated with Anatomical Areas

Six anatomical areas seen on the CC view are the locations for most radiographic abnormalities that can be identified on this view (Figure 11-16):

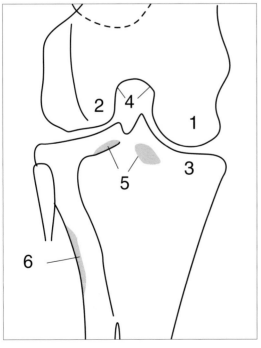

Figure 11-16. Most of the radiographic abnormalities that can be identified on the CC view occur at six anatomical locations. These are:
1. Medial femoral condyle
2. Lateral femoral condyle
3. Medial tibial condyle
4. Intercondylar fossa of the femur
5. Attachment sites for the cranial ligaments of the menisci
6. Lateral metaphyseal cortex of the proximal tibia
Secondary joint disease of the medial femorotibial joint will be demonstrated in Figure 11-26.

A. Medial Femoral Condyle

1) Subchondral lucent area in the center of the medial condyle. The lucent area can vary from shallow to deep (Figure 11-17).
2) The contour of the subchondral bone may appear flattened or interrupted by the lucency.
3) Periarticular productive change.

Radiographic Conclusions/Impressions
- Subchondral cyst*: Signs 1 and 2
- Secondary Joint Disease: Sign 3

B. Lateral Femoral Condyle

1) Subchondral lucent area of varying depths usually located more axially on the condyle.
2) Changes are uncommon when compared to the medial femoral condyle.

Radiographic Conclusions/Impressions
- Subchondral cyst: Sign 1

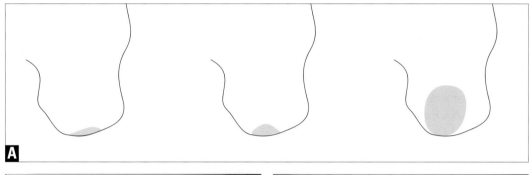

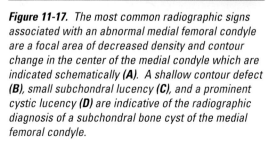

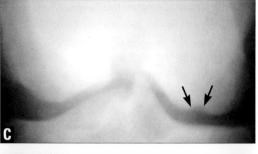

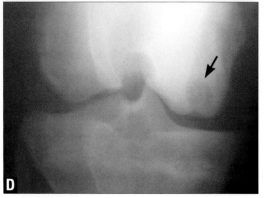

Figure 11-17. The most common radiographic signs associated with an abnormal medial femoral condyle are a focal area of decreased density and contour change in the center of the medial condyle which are indicated schematically *(A)*. A shallow contour defect *(B)*, small subchondral lucency *(C)*, and a prominent cystic lucency *(D)* are indicative of the radiographic diagnosis of a subchondral bone cyst of the medial femoral condyle.

Radiographic Interpretation of the Stifle and Proximal Tibia

* This term describes the radiographic finding and not the specific cause. A subchondral bone cyst refers to a solitary lucent lesion that may result from osteochondrosis or other developmental orthopedic disease, a bone infection earlier in life, or other known condition.

C. Medial Tibial Condyle

1) Lucent subchondral area similar to medial femoral condyle but occurring less frequently (Figure 11-18).
2) Focal subchondral sclerosis.
3) Periarticular productive change. This change is seen on the tibia before the femur.

Radiographic Conclusions/Impressions

- Subchondral cyst lesion: Signs 1 and 2
- Secondary joint disease: Sign 3

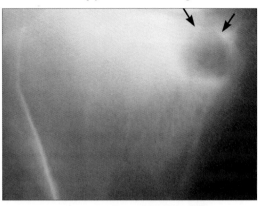

Figure 11-18. *A subchondral cystic lesion of the medial tibial condyle is seen infrequently. This cystic lesion has a suspected interruption in the subchondral bone (arrowheads) suggestive of a communication between the cavity of the cystic lesion and medial femorotibial joint. The prominent sclerotic rim is attributed to the pressure of the joint fluid communicating with the cystic area.*

D. Intercondylar Fossa of the Femur

1) Abnormal contour and decreased density to the medial "wall" of the intercondylar fossa (caudal cruciate ligament attachment).
2) Abnormal contour and decreased density to the lateral "wall" of the intercondylar fossa (cranial cruciate ligament attachment).
3) Radiodense body in the intercondylar fossa (Figure 11-19).
4) Periarticular productive change on axial aspect of the medial condyle.

Radiographic Conclusions/Impressions

- Fibro-osseous remodeling secondary to cranial cruciate (lateral wall) or caudal cruciate (medial wall) ligament damage: Signs 1 and 2
- Avulsion fracture from the tibial plateau: Sign 3
- Secondary joint disease: Sign 4

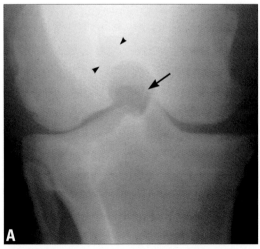 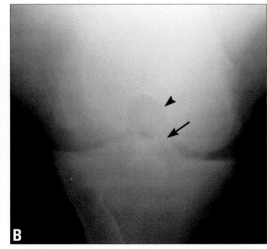

Figure 11-19. *The intercondylar fossa of the femur must be examined carefully on the CC view for evidence of a dense body indicative of an avulsion fracture (A). The decreased density in the lateral wall of the intercondylar fossa (arrowheads) is compatible with damage to the origin of the cranial cruciate ligament. The origin of the fracture (arrow) usually cannot be identified unless the fracture fragment (arrowhead) is large (B).*

E. Tibial Plateau

1) Lucent oval-shaped areas near midline, more commonly seen medially than laterally (Figure 11-20).
2) A sclerotic rim tends to surround the lucent areas in the chronic stage.
   Note: The lucent areas are confirmed to be located cranially on the tibial plateau by identification on the LM view (see Figure 11-15).
3) A focal lucency located lateral to the tibial spine is seen with injury at the insertion of the cranial cruciate ligament. This lucency is located more caudally than that for the cranial ligaments of the menisci and cannot be seen on the routine LM view.

Radiographic Conclusions/Impressions

- Fibro-osseous remodeling secondary to damage at the insertion of the cranial ligaments of the menisci or cranial cruciate ligament: Signs 1, 2, and 3

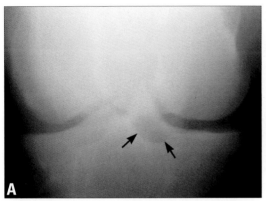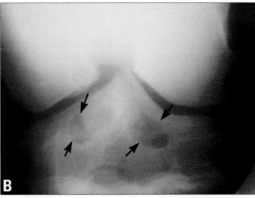

Figure 11-20. An oval-shaped lucency of the tibial plateau is identified more commonly medial to midline on the CC view *(A)* resulting from remodeling at the insertion of the cranial ligament of the medial meniscus. This remodeling change can also involve the cranial ligament of both menisci *(B)*. There is increased density associated with the lucency at the attachment site of the cranial ligament of the lateral meniscus. The lucency and productive remodeling changes were also identified on the LM view of this horse (see Figure 11-15) which confirms that the radiographic signs involved the areas of insertion of the cranial ligaments of the menisci.

F. Lateral Metaphyseal Region of the Tibia

There are three clinical conditions that are seen radiographically on the CC view associated with the lateral metaphyseal region of the proximal tibia. These are: incomplete fracture of the tibia, transverse linear lucency of the fibula, and soft tissue calcification.

Radiographic Signs Involving the Lateral Tibial Cortex

1) Periosteal reactive bone located 7 to 11 cm distal to the articular surface of the lateral condyle of the tibia (Figure 11-21).
2) Oblique lucent line associated with the periosteal reaction may be identified.
3) In chronic stages the bone of the lateral tibia appears sclerotic.
4) The lesion may be bilateral. A CC view of the contralateral limb is indicated.

Radiographic Conclusions/Impressions:

- Incomplete fracture: Signs 1-4

Radiographic Signs Involving the Fibula

The fibula can be seen on the CC view in this anatomical location and a transverse, lucent line can frequently be identified in it. This finding is commonly a result of incomplete ossification and represents an incidental finding. However, the periosteal surface of the bone proximal and distal to this linear lucency must be examined for periosteal reaction which is compatible with a fracture (Figure 11-21E).

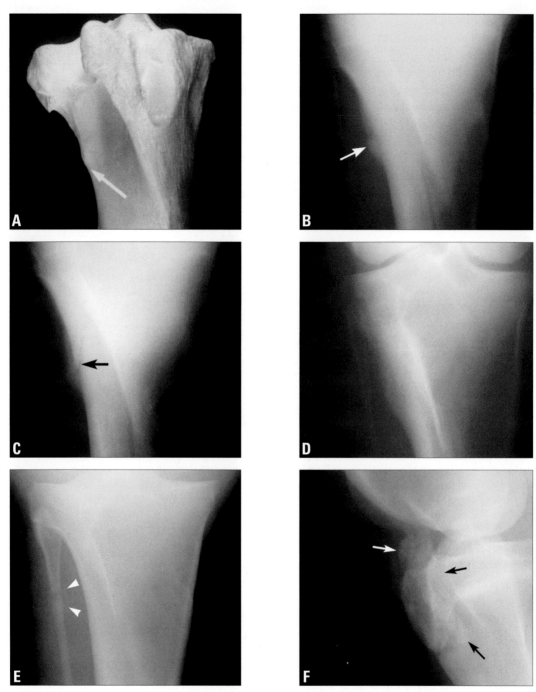

Figure 11-21. *Incomplete fractures are seen at the lateral metaphyseal area of the proximal tibia on the CC view. The center of the lesion is approximately 8.5 cm from the articular surface of the lateral condyle of the tibia (A). This lesion is identified by a focal periosteal reaction (B) with (C) or without an oblique fracture in the underlying cortex. The fracture line when identified extends from the cortical surface in the proximo-axial direction. In the chronic stages, a large, smooth callus can be identified (D). In this anatomical area, a transverse lucent line may be seen in the fibula which indicates incomplete ossification and this finding is usually without clinical significance. The exception (E) is a transverse lucent line that has an associated callus (arrowheads). Tumoral calcinosis is seen in the soft tissues in the muscular sulcus between the fibula and site of fractures of the lateral metaphyseal cortex of the tibia on the CC view, but it can also be seen extending more proximally (arrows) on the LM view (F).*

Radiographic Signs Involving Soft Tissue Calcification

In this anatomical area and proximally, soft tissue calcification is infrequently seen. The calcification tends to be located more proximal than the incomplete fractures of the tibia and fibula described previously, and may extend above the level of the tibial condylar surface (Figure 11-21F). This dystrophic calcification may be linear or large and rounded. It is located in the muscular sulcus associated with the tendons of the long digital extensor and peroneus tertius. The term "tumoral calcinosis" has been used to describe the lesion when the calcification is large and rounded. Clinical signs associated with this lesion vary from none to an abnormal gait characterized by a "swinging out" of the limb landing on the lateral part of the hoof wall. If there is an absence of clinical signs, conservative treatment is indicated. Surgical removal of the calcification is indicated if producing clinical signs, but the surgery can be difficult when there is extension of the lesion into the femorotibial joint capsule.

3. Lateral Oblique View: Radiographic Signs Associated with Anatomical Areas

This view supplements the CC view for very large horses because it permits the medial femoral condyle to be carefully evaluated (Figure 11-22 A). It also supplements the LM view for interpretation of the lateral ridge of the trochlea of the femur.

A. Medial Femoral Condyle

1) Loss of normal contour to the subchondral bone of the femoral condyle varying from a flattening to a shallow indentation to a cavitary lesion.
2) Subchondral lucent lesion (Figure 11-22 B).
3) Periarticular productive change on the caudolateral aspect of the medial condyle of the tibia.

Radiographic Conclusions/Impressions
- Subchondral cyst: Signs 1 and 2
- Secondary joint disease: Sign 3

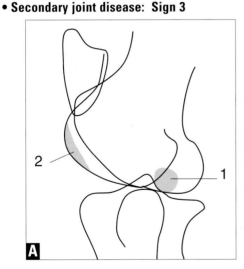

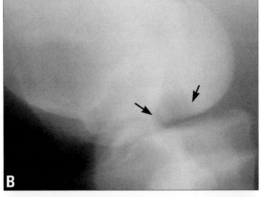

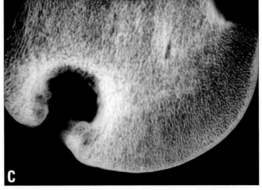

Figure 11-22. *The lateral oblique view **(A)** of the stifle is taken primarily to evaluate the medial femoral condyle (1) and lateral ridge of the femoral trochlea (2). The loss of the normal contour of the medial femoral condyle with subchondral lucency is indicative of a subchondral cyst **(B and C)**.*

B. Lateral Ridge of the Trochlea of the Femur

1) Loss of normal contour of the subchondral bone (Figure 11-23).
2) Decrease density to subchondral bone associated with the contour loss.
3) Sclerosis surrounding the area of subchondral bone loss and contour abnormality.
4) Radiodense bodies associated with the area of contour and density changes.
5) Dense bodies distal to the area with changes in contour and bone density. These bodies tend to enlarge and increase in density with chronicity because they embed in the synovium and grow.

Radiographic Conclusions/Impressions

• Osteochondrosis of the lateral ridge of the femor trochlea: Signs 1, 2, and 3
• Osteochondritis dissecans: Signs 4 and 5

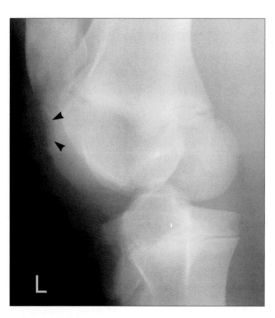

Figure 11-23. This lateral oblique view permits the soft tissue swelling of the femoropatellar joint and bony changes in the lateral ridge of the trochlea to be evaluated, supplementing findings seen with the LM view. A contour defect, underlying decreased bone density, and surrounding sclerosis can be seen (arrowheads). The LO view often provides additional information concerning the presence of fragmentation at the lesion site.

4. Patellar Skyline View: Radiographic Signs Associated with Anatomical Areas

A. Body and Non-Articular (Free) Surface of the Patella (Figure 11-24)

1) Sagittal linear lucent change.
2) Displaced body from the medial angle.
3) Productive response on the dorsolateral surface.

Radiographic Conclusions/Impressions

• Incomplete fracture: Sign 1
• Complete fracture: Sign 2
• Enthesophytosis at attachment of the biceps femoris and/or lateral patellar ligament: Sign 3

B. Articular Surface of the Patella (Figure 11-25)

1) Interruption of the normal contour more commonly seen at the medial part.
2) Subchondral bone loss surrounded by sclerosis.

Radiographic Conclusions/Impressions

• Complete fracture: Sign 1
• Subchondral cyst and secondary joint disease: Sign 2

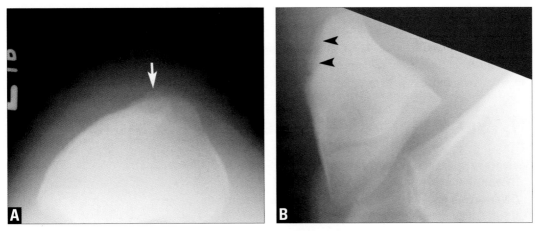

Figure 11-24. *Soft tissue swelling and a minor degree of productive bony response on the dorsolateral surface of the patella can be identified on the patellar skyline view (A). This reactive bone is seen on the dorsal surface of the patella in the area of attachment of the lateral patellar ligament (B).*

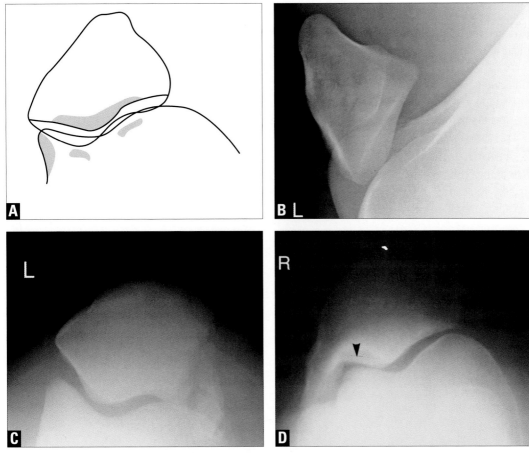

Figure 11-25. *Bony change at the articular surface of the patella can best be visualized on the patellar skyline (A). A fracture of the patella was suspected on the LM view (B), but the patellar skyline (C) permitted more detailed evaluation. A comminuted, complete fracture of the medial angle of the patella with patellar subluxation can be identified on the skyline view. Subchondral lucency (arrowhead) surrounded by sclerosis was identified in another horse with femoropatellar effusion (D). There is extensive, chronic productive change at the lateral angle of the patella which could not be completely evaluated on the LM view (see Figure 11-13 B).*

C. Trochlear Ridges and Subchondral Bone of the Femur
    1) Decreased subchondral density.
    2) Loss of normal contour to the abaxial aspect of the lateral ridge.
  Radiographic Conclusions/Impressions
    • Osteochondrosis with or without secondary joint disease: Signs 1 and 2

III. Secondary Joint Disease of the Stifle

Radiographic signs of secondary joint disease (SJD) of the stifle are:
    1) Periarticular productive change
    2) Narrowing of the joint space with subchondral sclerosis
    3) Soft tissue calcification
Radiographic signs of SJD are identified best on the CC and LO views when the medial femorotibial (FT) joint is involved and on the LM when the femoropatellar (FP) joint is involved.

1. Femorotibial Joint
SJD of the femorotibial joints occurs primarily at the medial FT joint and is first identified radiographically on the CC and LO as a periarticular remodeling of the medial tibial plateau. As remodeling changes progress, the distomedial aspect of the femur will have periarticular osteophytes. Small osteophytes may also be seen on the axial periarticular margin of the medial femoral condyle (Figure 11-26).

Narrowing of the joint space is seen best on the CC view (Figure 11-26 B). This finding is indicative of damage to the meniscus. Subchondral sclerosis is a common accompanying radiographic sign. Chronic injury to the meniscus can lead to calcification of the meniscus (Figure 11-26 C).

2. Femoropatellar Joint
SJD of the FP joint is identified on the LM view as periarticular remodeling at the apex and base of the patella. Radiographic signs of SJD of the femoropatellar joint space are more commonly seen first at the apex. In severe cases of FP joint disease, the basilar region is involved (see Figure 11-13 B).

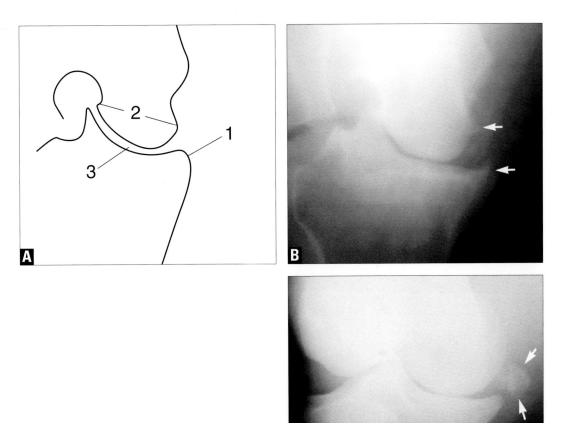

Figure 11-26. *Radiographic signs of severe secondary joint disease of the stifle are commonly seen on the CC view **(A)**. Signs seen at the medial femorotibial joint occur as periarticular osteophytes at the proximal tibia (1) followed by similar changes at the abaxial and axial margins of the medial femoral condyle (2). Joint space narrowing indicates medial meniscal damage (3). Prominent periarticular osteophytes (arrows) are seen at the proximomedial tibia and distomedial femur **(B)**. The narrowing of the medial femorotibial joint space and the soft tissue calcification (arrows) seen on the LO view **(C)** indicate that the secondary joint disease is secondary to severe medial meniscal injury followed by dystrophic calcification.*

NOTES

NOTES

NOTES

Chapter 12

The Role of Radiology in the Equine Purchase Examination

I. Introduction

Radiology plays an important role in equine purchase examinations. There are three major reasons a radiographic examination is included with purchase evaluation. The reasons are:
- To further evaluate a finding determined by a clinical examination.
- A screening technique for horses without clinical evidence of an abnormality.
- Seller wants to know if radiographic evidence of bone or joint disease exists prior to sale.

The seller often wants this latter determination for establishing a selling price and as an aid to negotiation.

Radiographic examinations are more disconcerting than other equine examination procedures, e.g., cardiac, ophthalmologic, lung auscultation, etc. This is true because the radiographic examination produces a permanent record (radiographs) which can be evaluated retrospectively. This radiographic review can determine three important features. These features include: 1) were the radiographs of diagnostic quality? 2) were adequate views taken to sufficiently examine the anatomical region in question? and 3) was the radiographic examination correctly interpreted? Therefore, technical quality pitfalls must be avoided.

Technical quality pitfalls associated with equine purchase examinations are:
- Overexposure
- Improper positioning
- Dark room errors
- Motion and preparation artifacts
- Insufficient identification of radiographs

Identification information is a very common pitfall and should include all of the following details:
- Name of the horse and owner
- Date of the radiographic examination
- Anatomical designations: right or left, front or hind, medial or lateral

Information to avoid these pitfalls should be permanently incorporated into the radiograph at time of exposure or during development. The use of one-inch tape as an "add-on" method of identification should be avoided in equine radiography in general but especially for purchase work.

The details associated with the adequate number of views for a routine examination of an anatomical region was provided previously. The anatomical regions commonly radiographed as part of purchase examinations and the recommended number of views for these routine examinations are:
- Distal extremity examination (5)
- Metacarpophalangeal (5)
- Tarsus (4)
- Stifle (3)

II. Avoiding Problems with Radiology

There are several general issues besides those discussed with quality, completeness of an examination, interpretation, and technical pitfalls associated with purchase evaluation. These issues have resulted in litigation so they must be reviewed.

1. **Value of the Horse Compared to the Cost of the Radiographic Examinations**
   The veterinarian's responsibility is to advise the client that radiographs can reveal valuable information that would allow them to provide better medical advice. The buyer can then accept or decline the radiographic examinations. My experience has demonstrated that the veterinarian who does not offer radiographic examinations to a client who is purchasing an "inexpensive" horse is making a serious mistake. A few buyers have brought litigation against the veterinarian alleging if they had been advised a better decision could have been possible with radiographic information, they would have certainly considered such examinations. Therefore, the veterinarian should write in the record that radiographic examinations were recommended, but the buyer declined radiographic examinations to avoid additional costs.

2. **Remembering Who the Veterinarian Works For – The Buyer, Seller, or Both?**
   Who does the veterinarian work for – the buyer, seller, or both? The situation a veterinarian must avoid is working as an agent for both the buyer and seller. It is advised that fewer problems occur when the veterinarian is the agent of the buyer.

3. **Utilization of the Radiographs by Others**
   The radiographs produced in the purchase examination are a part of the medical record and belong to the veterinarian conducting the examinations. The utilization of these radiographs by others, e.g., the seller, other buyers or veterinarians, requires the permission of the individual(s) who paid for the radiographic examination. It is recommended that such permission be written and retained as part of the veterinarian's record.

4. **Making Your Role as the Veterinarian Known to the Buyer**
   The veterinarian's opinion is given based on knowledge of the clinical history, patient evaluation supplemented by radiographic findings, and aided by knowledge of future athletic demands.

   A. **The Buyer Must Make the Purchase Decision Based on the Veterinarian's Opinion Plus Knowledge of the Athletic Demands expected, Cost, and Other Personal Factors**

   B. **The Veterinarian Must Beware**
   1. **If the Buyer's Expectations Are:**
      - A guarantee for future soundness
      - An appraisal of ability
      - An appraisal of the selling price
      - Future resale potential
   2. **If the Seller's Expectations Are:**
      - The veterinarian understands there is a lack of perfection in all horses
      - A quick examination
      - No interference with the sale
      - The veterinarian assumes responsibility for the condition of the horse.

III. Creating a Radiographic Report

The objective of the radiographic examination is to provide medical information that will assist in the decision to purchase or reject the horse. A radiographic report is an important part to this process. The veterinarian must carefully review all the radiographs and determine if the radiographic examination is of diagnostic quality, then assimilate the radiographic information in a logical manner (notes) to develop a report. In this process of identifying the radiographic signs, it is important to prioritize the findings from more significant to less significant to incidental findings. The radiographic conclusions and impressions are then established. It is extremely important that the veterinarian carefully explain to the client that radiographs **do not** reveal all abnormalities.

IV. When Should the Purchase Radiographs be Referred for Interpretation?

Referrals for radiographic interpretation are highly variable with veterinarians but there seems to be three conditions that result in referral that have been sent to me:
1. A need for additional expertise.
2. A controversy between two veterinarians resulting from differing interpretations.
3. An insurance company or an attorney requesting an expert opinion.

Some veterinarians routinely seek additional expertise with their purchase examinations. Often the purchase price of the horse these veterinarians are dealing with is high. These veterinarians say it is an "insurance" policy for them because the diagnostic quality, positioning, and interpretation of the radiographic examinations will be documented. In addition, the cost for the referral is passed directly to their client and the client usually seems satisfied with additional expertise in their decision-making process.

The second scenario for referral is when a controversy exists between two veterinarians resulting from differing opinions regarding interpretation of radiographic examinations. Multiple examination dates are commonly involved in these controversies. The veterinarian interpreting radiographs at a later date tends to have a major advantage because earlier suspected findings are more evident and additional findings tend to be identifiable due to remodeling changes. The expert must be very careful, and I have found the best guiding principle to be . . . "Make sure one's opinion is based on the radiographic signs identified on the radiographs taken at the time of each examination."

The third scenario involving insurance companies and attorneys is usually a result of an unresolved controversy. It has been my experience that the attorneys will want expert opinion on three questions. The first, "Are the radiographs diagnostic quality?" Second, "Is the examination complete?" And finally, "Did the veterinarian accurately interpret the radiographs?" The attorney for the plaintiff will be most interested in the first two questions, and the defense tends to be most interested in the conclusions and impressions expressed in the interpretation.

V. Where Can Expertise be Found to Refer Purchase Radiographic Examinations?

Expertise for interpreting purchase radiographs can be found in several locations. The more common sources are regional practitioners with interest in radiology, private specialty practices dealing with lameness, university clinics, and diplomates of the American College of Veterinary Radiology. There are advantages and disadvantages to each source so the practitioner must explore each to find the best working relationship. It is also important to determine if the expertise should be local, regional, or national.

VI. How Should a Veterinarian Respond if Threatened with Litigation?

Contact your malpractice insurance carrier and attorney IMMEDIATELY. While waiting to receive direction from these contacts, the following are important actions suggested:
1. **Volunteer no information either to the buyer or seller.**
2. **Release no radiographs or records related to the patient.**
3. **Gather all radiographs and records dealing with the patient and store them in a safe place.**
4. **Write down your recollection of events concerning the patient in question.**
5. **Keep a log of all follow-up events related to this patient.**

It is important to remember in dealing with potential litigation that you must remain isolated from the buyer and seller until you receive advice from your attorney.

I want to thank you for the opportunity to share my experiences with equine radiology and wish you great success in your future endeavors with purchase examinations. However, you should be alerted to the word "success." "Success is that place in the road where preparation and opportunity meet. But too few people recognize it because it comes disguised as sweat and hard work." – Anonymous.

NOTES

NOTES

NOTES

NOTES

INDEX

Page numbers followed by a *t* indicate a table;
page numbers followed by a *f* indicate a figure.